WHOLE

HEALTH

DENTISTRY

WHOLE
HEALTH
DENTISTRY

WHY YOUR MOUTH
IS THE KEY TO
YOUR BODY'S HEALTH

NAMRITA SINGH, DMD

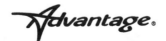

Published by Advantage, Charleston, South Carolina.
Member of Advantage Media Group.

ADVANTAGE is a registered trademark and the Advantage colophon is a trademark of Advantage Media Group, Inc.

Printed in the United States of America.

ISBN: 978-159932-360-2
LCCN: 2013936868

This publication is designed to provide accurate and authoritative information in regard to the subject matter covered. It is sold with the understanding that the publisher is not engaged in rendering legal, accounting, or other professional services. If legal advice or other expert assistance is required, the services of a competent professional person should be sought.

Advantage Media Group is proud to be a part of the Tree Neutral® program. Tree Neutral offsets the number of trees consumed in the production and printing of this book by taking proactive steps such as planting trees in direct proportion to the number of trees used to print books. To learn more about Tree Neutral, please visit www.treeneutral.com. To learn more about Advantage's commitment to being a responsible steward of the environment, please visit www.advantagefamily.com/green

Advantage Media Group is a leading publisher of business, motivation, and self-help authors. Do you have a manuscript or book idea that you would like to have considered for publication? Please visit www.amgbook.com or call 1.866.775.1696

DEDICATION

A wise man once said,
*"The child is like a river and his/her parents are the banks
along the side that guide the river on its path."*

For my parents,
whose guidance, encouragement and unshakable faith
led me down the path to endeavor the writing of a book.

For my children, Anika and Aman,
who were so very patient while I worked on this book.
Their faith in me is my inspiration. When I hear them tell their
friends that their mom is the best dentist in the world,
it makes me want to be the best, just for them.

For my staff and my team
who help me to be the dentist I want to be.
They gladly embrace every innovative idea I introduce in my
practice, knowing it will add hours of training to their already
hectic schedules. They do it because they believe in me,
and believe in giving the best quality of care for our patients.

TABLE OF CONTENTS

47 CHAPTER THREE

SLEEP APNEA

CHAPTER FOUR

PATIENT FAQs:

INTRODUCTION

I HAVE NOT ALWAYS BEEN IN LOVE WITH MY PRO-FESSION, but today I am proud to say that I am totally, unequivocally, and passionately devoted to it. It is a profession that allows me to contribute to people living long, healthy lives and to make them smile with confidence.

When something you love is attacked, you rise to its defense. If I had a penny for every time I heard, "I hate going to the dentist," I would be rich. These days, I am not as offended by such statements as I am curious about why people hold such negative opinions; after all, things have changed so much. I have been making an informal survey of people that I meet – at parties, at my kids' school events, or at the mall – and I have been asking each of them, "What's your opinion about going to the dentist? How much value do you put on your dental care?" From their answers, I have realized that most people have very little awareness of the necessity of routine dental checkups; they have many misconceptions about dental health; and they have no sense of urgency in completing basic treatments, like cleanings and fillings. Some of them have had painful previous dental experiences, and fear has prevented them from going back to the dentist. Some did not understand why they should go see the dentist regularly because, as they said, "nothing hurts." Some said dentists over-diagnosed conditions, so they did not trust dentists in general. Going to the dentist is expensive, and many people say they have other, more important things to do with their money. People's answers separated them into four categories. Most of the people I spoke with fell into three different categories: fearful, procrastinatory, and skeptical. The fourth and smallest group was made up of what I would call my ideal patients.

For the fearful, here is a story that might help you overcome your feelings.

People ask me why I decided to be a dentist, and I tell them I did not. My father decided for me. Right after I finished high school, my parents deposited me outside the dorm at a dental school in India. They expected me to come out a dentist 5 years later. Before I went to dental school, I had my first dental checkup. I was 17 years old. I got two fillings with no anesthesia. They were not small fillings; they were craters. I cried through my appointment, and I swore I would never go back. That was my introduction to dentistry. I am still dental-phobic. To this day, every time I see any anti-anxiety, non-pain-causing technology at a seminar or a meeting, I will get it for my practice. My first experience with dentistry became my first lesson. My mission as a dentist became making dental visits as pleasant and painless as possible for my patients. Because of advances in technology ranging from early diagnosis, which helps with minimally invasive dentistry, to various sedation and anxiety-reducing methods, the fearful can truly leave their fear behind now.

For those who are procrastinators, and think dentistry is not important, I have a message for you: I believe that you are avoiding taking care of your health and are really putting yourself at risk. My hope is that after you have read this book, you will see the dentist as an extension of your primary care physician; I hope you will understand that what a dentist sees in your mouth reflects what is going on in the rest of your body and that your oral conditions can impact your overall health.

Take the most common symptom: bleeding gums. The mouth-related diagnosis for such a symptom could be poor oral hygiene, improper brushing and/or flossing, gingivitis, or periodontitis. Overall health conditions in the body that can cause the same symptoms could be poor nutrition, vitamin deficiencies, uncontrolled diabetes, and hypertension. This symptom could also be a side effect of blood-pressure medication, anti-seizure medication, blood thinners, or physiologic conditions, such as pregnancy.

Now, let's look at the dangers of bleeding gums. Bleeding gums can lead to the following conditions: progressively severe periodontal disease; loss of the supporting jawbone; loose or missing teeth; a poor bite, which leads to poor nutrition; or a smile that you would not feel good about. On the systemic side, the dangers of not treating bleeding gums could lead to harmful bacteria from the mouth entering the bloodstream, reaching other parts of the body, and causing a variety of problems: digestive system disorders, respiratory problems, heart attacks, strokes, poorly controlled diabetes, preterm pregnancy, underweight babies, or cancer. The list goes on and on. Three out of four Americans have some sort of periodontitis. These individuals are all at some risk of contracting any of these other conditions. If you are a procrastinator, ask yourself this: Is your health so unimportant to you that you would continue to put it on the back burner because you are so busy?

For the skeptics, those who believe that dentists over-diagnose in order to make money, realize that the world as you know it has changed drastically over the last two decades – and so has dentistry. Just as my kids will probably never know what it would be like to live without a phone on which they can e-mail, talk, and text at the same time, the new generation of dental patients will most likely never see an amalgam filling that contains mercury. Practitioners have introduced new technology and materials, and this introduction has changed the practice of dentistry. Practitioners have made tremendous advances in diagnostic tests. As a patient, you have a right to be informed. Ask your dentist why he or she is recommending a course of treatment. Is there an alternative treatment plan? Each part of your treatment can be explained in layman's terms. A skeptic should have no reason to stay a skeptic once he or she is educated. This book is for you skeptics in particular; once you are informed, you will understand your dentist's recommendations.

This book is also for you, my ideal patient, because nobody knows everything. I wish I could sit with every patient for hours and explain every new treatment that the field of dentistry now offers. Instead, that information is here, in this book, for you. Whether your challenges include snoring, sleep apnea, or temperomandibular disorders (TMD) that lead to migraines or headaches, you can find resolution: all these conditions may now be treated by your dentist.

It is my hope that through this book I can make you more aware and more open to all that is available to you, so that you can become an ideal patient: a fearless, well-informed consumer and an advocate for your own health.

~ Namrita Singh

CHAPTER ONE

YOUR MOUTH IS THE WINDOW TO YOUR HEALTH

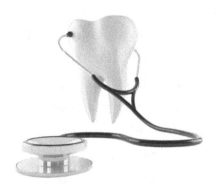

YOU WALK INTO MY OFFICE AND TAKE A SEAT. I ask, "What brings you in today?" Nine times out of ten, you say, "I just came for my regular cleaning." When I hear that, all I can do is look at you and wonder if you know how much of the big picture you are missing. If you think that a regular cleaning is mainly what your dentist can and should do for you, you are really shortchanging yourself.

Now, there is nothing wrong with wanting a dental cleaning. I am glad you want one. You have a definite advantage over the person who, for whatever reason, has not had a dental cleaning for years. However, a dental cleaning is treatment rendered under the care of a licensed dentist after he or she makes a diagnosis regarding the healthy or diseased status of your teeth and gums. Based on that diagnosis, the type of treatment the dentist will recommend could range from *prophylaxis*, which is preventative gum therapy, to scaling, root cleaning, or more extensive gum therapy. Any other kind of dental cleaning is the one performed by you, using a toothbrush, toothpaste, and floss.

About 80 percent of America's adult population has some form of gum disease. Children can get gum disease as well. Dentists can assess the risk of *periodontal disease* in both children and adults by using oral DNA tests that detect and measure the levels of specific pathogenic bacteria that cause periodontal disease.

By all means, come to the dentist and ask for a cleaning, but wait for the diagnosis and get the recommended gum therapy according to that diagnosis. Your gums' health, or what we call "periodontal health," does not depend on your age or level of home care. It also does not depend on what your insurance covers. If you have questions about how or why a dentist makes a diagnosis, find a dentist who will show you the evidence in an objective, measurable manner that you can understand.

A mouth is important, even from a child's perspective. For instance, it is easy for my eight-year-old son to answer when I ask him, "What do you do with your mouth?"

"I eat with it," he says. "I drink with it. I speak. I smile."

The problem is that most of us see the mouth and its health as a separate entity from the rest of the body. That so many of us consider oral health as something apart from the rest of our physical health may have its roots in how physicians are schooled. While cardiologists specialize in hearts and ENT surgeons see the ear, nose, and throat, these cardiologists and surgeons all can be classified as physicians, and they start out with a common education before choosing a specialty. People go to primary care physicians to get an examination of the entire body; then, when and if the primary care physician deems it necessary, a patient goes to a specialist for consultation on a certain body part that needs more attention.

Dentists fall into a different category. Our education is more specific to the mouth, the teeth, the jaws, and the adjacent structures. General dentists, like myself, are primary care dentists; we refer patients to other dental specialists if the necessary treatment or procedures are beyond our scope of practice. Because dentists practice separately in this category, the average patient not only separates dentists from other healthcare providers and physicians, but also disconnects oral health and general health.

I want to emphasize that although the mouth is a vital, sensitive, and complicated organ that requires its own specialization, it is still a part of the body. Consider its anatomical position in relation to other adjacent structures. It is right next to the most important sensory organs: eyes, ears, and nose. It gives residence to the tongue, without which a person could not speak, taste, or swallow. It is the entryway into the body for nutrition, and it is the gateway to the airway. An abscess in the mouth can lead to difficulty in breathing (because it puts pressure on the airway), problems in eating or swallowing, or to infection of the eye, ear, nose, or brain. *A healthy mouth supports a healthy body and supports life.* A diseased mouth can affect any or all of the above functions and organs so vital to our lives, yet people do not take good care of their mouths. In a patient who has come in asking for a regular cleaning, I might see broken teeth, infected gums, or root abscesses. This patient, who would not ignore a little swelling on his toe for a single day, will live with rotting, abscessed teeth and bleeding gums for years. Why?

I see one of my old friends every month at our book club. This friend also happens to be a patient of mine. Each time I see her she says, "I've got to come in and get the crown done. The tooth you said was cracked hurts when I chew on it now." Because we are friends, I know her hesitation is not related to trust or a question of needing treatment. She knows what she needs to do, yet she has been putting it off for a year.

Is this hesitation a lack of knowledge, procrastination, or just plain denial? When I dig a little deeper, I find there are lots of reasons for hesitation, all very personal to each patient. They are afraid of the unknowns, from the amount of pain to the potential cost. People perceive dentistry as painful, expensive, and full of nasty surprises. While I will address these in later chapters, know for now that the fear of the unknown can easily be conquered by participating in an exchange of information and receiving knowledge of what to expect. Given all the technological advances in dentistry, fear of pain and any nagging anxiety over what has happened in the past should stay in the past. Dentists may not be able to help patients with their financial situations, but when we, as healthcare providers, see that an individual is a well informed and motivated patient, we will work with that individual to find a way to achieve a common goal, which is optimal dental health that goes beyond the mouth for a healthy person.

Statistics indicate that 20 percent of Americans see their dentists more regularly than their physicians. Dentists belong to the group of primary healthcare providers that see the same patients several times a year. We are those patients' first line of defense against any disease that has a correlation to the mouth. We can only fulfill that role if patients give us an opportunity to conduct a thorough, systematic examination – with the help of diagnostic aids and tests – in order to make a comprehensive evaluation of each individual patient. Then, we can recommend to each person the treatment that is customized to that individual's specific needs and that will get that patient's mouth and body in optimal health.

MULTI-ORGAN EFFECTS OF PERIODONTAL DISEASE

The list of other systems and organs in the body that can be adversely affected by the conditions in the mouth is a long one. My aim is not to present every single name on that list; the effects discussed in this section are just the tip of the iceberg. I want to show clearly how important dental health is for the rest of the body.

Let's start with the most common infection of the mouth: a gum infection. A gum infection is a symptom of periodontal disease, a chronic inflammatory disease linked to increased inflammation in the body. It reaches your bloodstream easily because it is a bacterial infection. The various systemic conditions associated with periodontal disease are the following: Type II Diabetes; cardiovascular disease; arteriosclerosis; vascular diseases, such as strokes; Alzheimer's disease; chronic respiratory diseases, like COPD (chronic obstructive pulmonary disease); osteoporosis; rheumatoid arthritis; pancreatic and kidney cancers; and blood cancers.

For example, diabetes creates a glucose level in the body that is not controlled. It lowers immunity, and it also causes increased sensitivity to certain stimuli to which one would not normally react. For instance, a normal person would experience some level of gum inflammation if he or she had calculus (calcified deposit of plaque) on his or her teeth. In a diabetic, developing *calculus* can cause the gums to react in a very exacerbated manner. *Hypertension* (high blood pressure) and diabetes both can cause a similar kind of inflammatory response to plaque and calculus in the gums. Dentists clinically observe the inflammatory response as swollen, discolored, and bleeding gums that cause bad breath. A dentist who spots the symptom of bleeding gums in a patient can screen for underlying medical conditions, like diabetes and hypertension, and refer that patient to his or her family physician in a timely manner.

Recording patients' vital signs is an important part of the dental examination. This includes checking patients' blood pressure. If the dentist notes repeated elevated blood-pressure recordings, the dentist will refer the patient to his or her physician. High blood pressure can cause many issues, such as strokes and heart attacks. People who do not know they have elevated blood pressure can be walking time bombs. Sudden cardiac death happens most often to people who have uncontrolled blood pressure – people who have not been on medication and have never been diagnosed.

For expectant mothers, developing periodontal disease can lead to low birth-weight and preterm babies. Infertility and erectile dysfunction syndrome are also associated with periodontal disease. Men with periodontal disease are 49 percent more likely to develop kidney cancer; they are 54 percent more likely to develop pancreatic cancer; and they are 30 percent more likely to develop blood cancer. Dental care is not just about removing plaque or getting a regular cleaning. Optimal periodontal treatment is necessary for overall health and wellbeing, and it might well save your life.

ORAL CANCERS

The next vital component of a dental exam is oral cancer screening. Oral cancer is routinely missed in a physical, but a dentist can use a range of technologies to detect any precancerous changes in the mucous membranes of the patient's mouth.

Oral cancers can develop in any part of the oral cavity or even in the oropharynx. Most of these cancers begin in the tongue or the floor of the mouth; however, such cancers can appear on any surface of the mouth, including the lips, cheek, or palate. Unfortunately, the cancer does not just stay where it starts; instead, oral cancer can spread and usually does so through the lymphatic system. Most of the lymph nodes are located right in the neck area, and the lymphatic system can spread these cancer cells to other organs, like the lungs or kidneys. If oral cancer is undiagnosed until the late stages, the mortality rate for patients who have had oral cancer for five years is about 45 percent.

SMOKING, DIPPING, DRUG ADDICTIONS, AND EATING DISORDERS

When dentists look in patients' mouths, we look for little bumps and swellings in the cheeks or any rough areas. The mouth can tell its own story about the patient. When dentists start asking patients, "Do you smoke? Do you dip? Do you have acid reflux? What is it that is causing these conditions in your mouth?," we often find that the patients' medical issues either have not been diagnosed or are not under control. People who have eating disorders, for example, might not be open to disclosing their situation in their medical history. When a dentist uses a high-magnification, intra-oral camera on such patients in order to show how their teeth have been eroded by acid, those patients are more likely to admit to the disorder and, possibly, even seek help.

The effects of smoking are evident on the teeth, as are those of chewing tobacco. When a dentist looks in a dipper's mouth and determines which side is used for dipping, the dipper is usually stunned. Usually, the dentist can determine this because he or she can see an ugly, white, corrugated patch that is probably precancerous. That is when the dentist will admonish the patient, "Did you know that one in five people die when they contract oral cancer? Is this a consequence you are ready to accept?"

Dentists see teenagers whose parents may not know that they smoke, but the dentists can tell; when dentists look in the mouths of these patients and say, "You are a smoker, and you need to quit," the teenagers are usually surprised and want to know how dentists know. The dentist's camera can easily display the black, tar-like stains on the inside of a smoker's teeth. The smokers might not be able to see the tar deposits in their lungs. They cannot see the abnormal cells that form tumors and eventually cause them to die. Yet, when dentists show them those stains on their teeth and say, "That's probably what's happening in your lungs," they get the picture. That is a visual which is difficult for the physician to show but very easy for the dentist to show. A number of patients I have treated in my practice, and who I identified as smokers, have come back to tell me, "I quit and haven't smoked for the last three months," or, "I haven't smoked for the last year." To me, that is very satisfying. I feel that somewhere along the way, I improved their quality of life; I helped their family and their children by helping these patients live longer and healthier.

That is the scope of dentistry. If people do not go to the dentist and do not get that check on their overall health, they would not know the consequences.

Drugs, too, leave their mark in the mouth. Methamphetamines, cocaine, and most street drugs have adverse effects on the teeth. They cause typical lesions in the mouth. The lesions are right next to the gums and show up as dark-brown spots, along with tooth decay, from one side of the mouth to the other. There is a term for this condition, in fact: *meth mouth*. Treating a mouth affected by drug addiction has its challenges, and the most important one is communicating with the patient about the underlying cause of the condition of his or her teeth. Ideally, that gives the dentist a pathway to talking with the patient about seeking drug rehabilitation. If nothing else, as dentists we can always appeal to a patient's vanity. Everybody wants to smile and look nice. If having brown, spotty, rotting, and missing teeth gets to someone, so be it. That can be the goad it takes to make the patient admit that he or she has a drug addiction and motivate him or her to get help.

It is also dentists' responsibility to share suspicions with patients' parents or legal guardians when we see an underage patient whose mouth shows evidence of drug use, smoking, or eating disorders. Often, the parents have had suspicions, too, but when they have clinical evidence to support their worries, they are in a better position to address this issue with their children.

CHAPTER TWO

A Healthy Bite for a Healthy Body:
THE NEUROMUSCULAR APPROACH

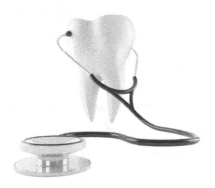

Perils of
Piecemeal Dentistry

A WISE MAN ONCE SAID, "THE LESS YOU KNOW, THE MORE EVERYTHING SEEMS NORMAL."

This is very true, especially when it comes to the bite. For a long time, I looked at teeth as thirty-two individual entities lined up in the upper and lower arches of the mouth, half next to each other and the other half opposing each other. The teeth obviously had to come together a certain way in order to allow chewing, swallowing, and talking. As a dentist, the designated savior of teeth, I felt that each tooth was sacred and had to be saved at any cost. If I saw a cavity, I knew it needed a filling. If I saw a fractured tooth, I knew it needed a crown or an extraction and an implant. To a large degree, my colleagues and I have all practiced dentistry in a piecemeal fashion. Sometimes, even when we see issues in adjacent teeth, our patients limit us by wanting to get only that one broken tooth fixed. People say things like, "Let's just do the one that is worst," or ask to have fixed the tooth that hurts the most.

Dentists listen to patients because we want to get patients out of pain and make them happy. However, the fact is that one healthy, painless, and strong tooth is not of much use without teeth on either side to support it or without any opposing it. A quarterback can do nothing without a linebacker or a runner. Your teeth are one organ, part of the craniomandibular system. This system includes not only the hard and soft tissue of the mouth, but the muscles, the jaws, the skull, and the nerves that innervate all these structures; all are a part of the craniomandibular system and work together. If any part of that system is in dysfunction in a patient, an expert must evaluate the entire system before reaching a diagnosis. Dentists look for certain indicators and signs that may not be causing problems to patients at the moment, but which can eventually lead to serious health issues. Dentists need to take preventative health measures before patients are faced with the related issues.

Overall, single-tooth dentistry really does not provide a reliable prognosis. For dentists to come to an accurate diagnosis and treat the mouth as a whole, it is necessary they have a more comprehensive approach to examination.

THE TOOTH TEAM:
THE CRANIOMANDIBULAR COMPLEX

We classify teeth into groups: incisors for cutting, cuspids for tearing, and premolars and molars for grinding. The tooth types all have their own specific functions. For patients, the knowledge of how these teeth come together in pairs to function or rest is very important, not only for the longevity of the restorations being placed in the mouth but also for the health of related structures affected by these functions, like the muscles, nerves, and joints. Besides gum infection and tooth decay, the most common cause of disease of the mouth is abnormal forces acting on the teeth. This is usually self-inflicted by habits like grinding or clenching. While the first two pathologies, gum infection and tooth decay, are relatively easier to diagnose and treat, abnormal forces leading to trauma to teeth is much more severe to treat; it needs to be managed in a timely, effective manner.

We live in a stressful world today, and I have seen the stress exhibit itself in my patients. When I look into people's mouths and see worn-down, fractured teeth, I usually ask them, jokingly, "Do you chew rocks?"

They reply, "No, but I've been stressed lately. I think I am grinding my teeth."

For the patients who think they grind or clench their teeth because of stress, I want to clarify that stress is a contributing factor, not the underlying cause of that habit. Most patients know that worn-down, flat, or saucer-shaped depressions on the chewing surface of the teeth may be a sign of grinding or clenching. What they do not know is that their grinding or clenching is usually a symptom of an unhealthy bite, or a *traumatic bite*. What they also may not know is that a receding gum line and the notching of the teeth they see at the area of gum recession is not because of using a hard toothbrush or conducting overzealous brushing. Those notches or *abfractions*, are symptomatic of a traumatic bite. Each tooth is the weakest at its neck, where the root of the tooth begins and the crown of the tooth narrows down. Abnormal forces applied to the teeth cause them to flex at the neck, which can produce fractures in that junction. These teeth are then at risk of fracturing completely at the gum line if the abnormal forces are not controlled.

THE TRAUMATIC BITE AND ITS EFFECTS

Usually, upper and lower teeth are separated at rest, while talking, and even while eating. They meet when people have to swallow; otherwise, people hardly ever hold the teeth together. People swallow about 2,000 times per day. A healthy bite is one that allows the muscles to stay in a state of relaxation during function and rest. An unhealthy or traumatic bite is one that has premature contact of teeth during closure or chewing. This habit sends a message to the muscles that are contracting to bring about the movement of the jaw to avoid those premature contacts, or to grind the teeth away in order to make the bite even and symmetrical again.

We can compare this to the idea of a man walking with a stone in one shoe. This man's tendency would be to avoid stepping down full force on the shoe with the stone in it, which automatically puts more pressure on the other foot, causing a limp. Over a period of time, the muscles of the leg bearing more pressure will be stiffer and the muscles of the leg not working at all will weaken. The pressure from the leg will transfer to the hip, because of the change in gait, and this will also eventually cause hip or lower back pain.

Similarly, the jaw muscles are in a state of asymmetrical contraction. The TMJ or temperomandibular joint are on each side of the jaw and work together to help the lower jaw move against the skull. The name comes from the two bones that help form the joint – the temporal bone which is part of the skull and the mandible or the lower jawbone. Between the two bones lies the articular disc. The underside of the disc mates with the part of the lower jaw called the condyle, and the upper side mates with the part of the temporal bone called the glenoid *fossa*.

Asymmetric forces on the temporomandibular joint can cause referred pain to the head and back muscles when there are premature contacts. An abnormal force that has caused a tooth to fracture can also cause a crown to fracture, or an implant to fail, if the force is not managed first.

In some cases, such as those in which teeth are affected by gum infection, patients already have compromised gum and bone support. Dentists need to protect such teeth from developing into a traumatic bite, since those teeth are already weak. While periodontal treatment can control or cure infection or inflammation, continued trauma will not allow the supporting structures (that is, the jawbone and gums) to heal completely or stabilize over a long time.

That is why checking the health of the bite is an important aspect of a comprehensive dental examination. It is significant in predicting the prognosis of restorative (fillings/crowns) and periodontal treatments (gum therapy), which are the main fields of dentistry. People go to the dentist to get fillings, or crowns, when they have broken a tooth or are suffering from decayed teeth. They go to the dentist because of a gum infection or because of symptoms like bad breath or bleeding gums. However, any related treatments cannot be effective until the dentists and patients have also managed the abnormal forces on those teeth.

MALOCCLUSION AND ITS CAUSES IN CHILDREN

The way the teeth come together is called *occlusion*. Surveys have shown that 80 percent of Americans have a "bad bite," or *malocclusion*. There are many possible causes for malocclusion in children: some sort of airway obstruction during a child's development period, or allergies to certain food types, environmental pollutants, pollen, and so forth. The normal way of breathing is through the nose. When a child has a stuffy or runny nose for prolonged periods of time, he or she starts breathing through the mouth. In that case, the nose cannot do its job of filtering environmental pollutants any more;

instead, the adenoids and the tonsils receive the pollutants and toxins inhaled along with the air. The adenoids and the tonsils get enlarged in order to fight these pollutants. That is a normal immunological reaction of the body meant for protection, but it closes the airways further and increases the risk of sleep apnea, which is a very serious condition, especially in children. I review sleep apnea in detail in the third chapter of this book, but there is such a strong correlation between grinding, TMJ disorders, and sleep apnea that I thought it should be mentioned here.

Now, let's look at how mouth breathing can cause bite and TMJ issues. During the stages of nasal breathing, the tongue rests against the palate. The outward pressure of the tongue from the inside balances the inward pressure of the cheek muscles from the outside. This creates a nice, U-shaped arch of teeth. During the stages of mouth breathing, the lower jaw comes down, and the tongue settles on the bottom teeth, to allow air to pass through the mouth and into the airway. With the outward force of the tongue out of the picture, there is no counteracting force to balance the inward force of the cheek muscles. This causes the arch of the teeth to constrict and become V-shaped, with less room for all the teeth to act in alignment. As the tongue rests on the lower molars, it prevents those molars from erupting completely; as a result, a mouth-breathing individual has to over-close the mouth to get his or her back teeth together. This creates an excessive overbite. As the bite is over-closed, the lower jaw is pushed back even more. The space for the tongue is decreased, so the tongue is forced to fall back, too. This causes more obstruction in the airway.

Thus, something that started as a reaction to simple, seasonal allergies for a prolonged period of time (one summer in a child's life), can actually make an individual a mouth-breather for life and create malocclusion in his or her mouth. In such a case, the abnormal position of the tongue causes an abnormal swallowing motion. The tongue pushes on the sides of the teeth and creates indentations in its lateral borders, known as *scalloped tongue*. This is what dentists look for during a comprehensive dental exam. Note that there is a 75 percent overlap between obstructive sleep apnea and craniomandibular disorders. An imbalance in muscular forces leads to abnormal pressure on the jawbone during development, which in turn causes a skeletal change. This change cannot be fixed dentally. It requires surgical intervention in adulthood. That is why it is so important to diagnose and correct these issues during the development stages in a child, while the child is still growing.

Another cause of this imbalance in children is beginning to bottle-feed a child too early in its infancy. Bottle-feeding requires a similar downward tongue position as that of a mouth breather; in contrast, breastfeeding requires the tongue to be up and raised toward the palate, which is the best position for development of balanced muscular forces.

A similar issue occurs with prolonged thumb sucking. When a child sucks his or her thumb, the thumb pushes the palate upward, and the upper teeth do not erupt downward because the thumb is in the middle of the mouth. This position causes an open bite, one in which the upper and lower teeth do not come together at all.

Malocclusion also happens to be a side effect of evolution. As humans have evolved into creatures with refined diets, our need for molars has diminished. People do not chew a great deal. Our jaw size is decreasing, but the number of teeth is still the same, which is why third molar (wisdom teeth) impactions are so common.

EFFECTS OF MALOCCLUSION
IN ADULTS

A traumatic bite can also be caused in adulthood. Baby boomers make up a large percentage of dental patients who require extensive dental work. They have had cavities that were filled with big silver fillings and then replaced; some fillings were replaced by porcelain crowns and some replaced by resin fillings. People may have a whole array of different dental materials in their mouths. The materials' rate of wear in the mouth is different, so a combination of materials can cause an uneven occlusal contact between teeth. Occlusal disharmony can cause the muscles to be in state of spasm or a hypertonic state. This disharmony can also cause the lower jaw to be pushed back, thereby causing the temperomandibular joint to be pushed backward in its fossa (the joint to be pushed backwards against the bone it's articulating with). In that case, abnormal pressure causes compression of the disc between the joint and the fossa, leading to irritation to the nerves present there, including the trigeminal; the irritation, in turn, causes pain. The trigeminal nerve is divided into three major branches that innervate the upper part of the head, the upper jaw and the teeth, and the lower jaw and the teeth. Any kind of irritation in any of these areas can cause referred pain, such as migraines, neck and shoulder pain, or even tingling in the hands and fingers.

Diagnosing Migraines

Let's talk about headaches and migraines in general. When patients come in to visit dentists, and we dentists see worn-down, broken teeth, there are many questions we may ask those patients that might seem completely unrelated to teeth:

- "Do you sleep well at night?"
- "Do you get up feeling well-rested in the morning?"
- "Do you snore?"

These questions pertain to sleep apnea, which is commonly associated with grinding and clenching habits. In the mouth, these habits are visible through worn-down, broken teeth. Then, we ask questions like the following:

- "Do your jaws hurt when you open and close your mouth?"
- "Are you having pain when chewing?"
- "Do you have any headaches, especially morning headaches?"
- "Do you have migraines?"

If the patients answer any of these questions in the affirmative, we ask them if they have had an MRI to diagnose migraines, or if they have seen a general physician, a neurologist, or (if relevant) a gynecologist. We also ask if the patients are on any medications and, if so, how effective the medications are.

An important part of the related examination is measuring the patient's normal range of motion in the muscles of the head and neck. We start with measuring the maximum range of the opening of the mouth, but we also measure the extension and flexion of the head and neck muscles. There is a normal or average range of opening of the mouth for a man and a woman; if a patient cannot open his or her mouth that wide, there is usually an underlying issue, either in the muscles or the joint itself. Know that malocclusion, premature contacts of teeth, spasms in jaw muscles, and TMJ pathology can all trigger the pain of migraines and headaches.

The treatment of your migraine or headaches might lie in the hands of your dentist, but it is possible that you are still totally unaware of this. It is fairly easy for a dentist trained in this field to validate if a patient's migraines and/or headaches indeed arise from an underling craniodental disharmony.

When dentists do come to that conclusion, we control the pain by reducing inflammation of the temperomandibular joint. Dentists do this by helping patients control the parafunctional habit causing the inflammation, all while making sure each patient's airway is maintained. As I discussed earlier, airway obstruction (that is, sleep apnea) is frequently connected to teeth grinding, or *bruxism*.

Pain in the neck or shoulders, and even arms can be triggered by TMD. Based on the results of a number of diagnostic tests, including some motor reflex and nerve tests, dentists can decide if the origin of the pain is primary (that is, if it is arising from the dentofacial complex), or if it is secondary. In the latter case, the dentist will refer the patient to a specific physician, neurologist, or chiropractor for treatment. Knowing the cause of the pain allows dentists to render therapy customized to each patient and his or her point of origin of the pain. Patients with secondary issues benefit from symptomatic treatment, like nighttime appliances that prevent grinding and clenching, until the time at which the right specialist can address their actual, underlying cause of pain.

Besides using reflex tests, dentists can also use something known as the Tech-Scan for a more detailed analysis of a patient's bite. A Tech-Scan is a pressure-mapping system that, along with other data, shows where a patient's teeth contact first and with how much pressure. This allows a dentist to see where to adjust or remove the premature contact in a patient's mouth.

TREATMENT MODALITIES FOR PAIN ARISING FROM TMD

After diagnosing a patient, usually a dentist fits a rehabilitative orthotic for that patient to wear for a certain period of time. During that period, the dentist provides the patient with adjunctive physical therapy. The orthotic prevents grinding of teeth, while the adjunctive therapy allows the muscles to relax and the TMJ (temporomandibular joint) to reposition; that way, there is no longer any pressure or irritation to the nerves surrounding the TMJ.

Dentists sometimes recommend both daytime and nighttime appliances for patients who have pain primarily originating from temperomandibular disorders – TMD. These appliances help to decompress the TMJ and reduce inflammation during both daytime and nighttime. Some patients clench and grind their jaws and teeth, respectively, during the day as well. A daytime appliance should be worn during the entire day, even at moments of eating and drinking. The appliance changes a patient's bite without that patient undergoing orthodontic movement or full-mouth rehabilitation with multiple crowns. After the patient wears the daytime appliance for twelve weeks, and the pain associated with inflammation is reduced to a minimum, the dentist leads the patient through a slow weaning process and reduces daytime appliance wear until the patient no longer needs to wear the appliance. Sometimes a patient may need a more permanent change through orthodontics or crowns to keep the new bite.

A whole host of other treatment modalities are based on specific patient needs for pain management. What is important to note is that if a traumatic bite is not addressed and treated, it can cause worn-down, broken teeth that are hard to restore until the cause is addressed and treated. For instance, a patient might either need implants or crowns, depending on the severity of the tooth fracture, and he or she might need root canals, if the nerves within the teeth gets inflamed due to trauma.

A traumatic bite can also cause a patient TMD-associated pain, which can result in headaches, migraines, and neck or shoulder pain. A patient may also experience other neuromuscular symptoms, like tingling or numbness of the hands; this connection is because the origination of the vascular circulation that goes into the extremities, like the hands, is located in the neck area. Another symptom could be ear pain, or ringing in the ears, because the ear is right next to the TMJ, and pressure in that area will cause irritation of the auricular nerve that goes into the ear.

APPLIANCE THERAPY
VERSUS STORE-BOUGHT
BITE SPLINTS

Most likely, some people have been grinding their teeth for twenty years. They might have significant tooth damage and need crowns. However, if they get crowns without fixing the underlying problem of grinding their teeth, they will destroy those crowns by grinding too, and their symptoms are going to stay the same. Most of the time, these patients know they grind their teeth at night. They say that they have already addressed the problem by buying a night guard, or a splint, on the Internet or at a pharmacy. These splints are usually thermoplastic; that is, they soften when immersed in hot water and harden in the mouth while cooling. These splints only put a plastic barrier in between the upper and lower teeth. A patient wearing such a splint might still be clenching or grinding, but instead of making tooth-to-tooth contact, he or she grinds on plastic. That does offer some protection to the teeth, but it does not address the underlying cause of the TMD at all. In fact, if the splint is too thick, it can reposition the jaw, thereby putting more pressure on the joint space. This additional pressure can exacerbate the TMD instead of alleviating the symptoms.

A dentist makes an orthotic for a patient by recording the patient's psysiological bite. This bite is the position of the lower jaw in relation to the upper jaw at the moment when the muscles of mastication are relaxed and the TMJ is situated in its joint space properly, the place where it exerts the least pressure on the disc. This is the most significant step in the fabrication of an orthotic appliance. A store-bought splint does not take this crucial step into account whatsoever.

BITE REGISTRATION

The procedure of recording a patient's bite so that a dentist can make an orthotic to replicate it is called *bite registration*. There are many different ways for a dentist to record this bite. They all involve putting a pliable dental material in between the patient's upper and lower teeth, and then having the patient keep his or her mouth closed in a certain position until the material hardens. That position of closure is what is most significant. A TMD patient already has tense muscles and pain in the jaw, so he or she will not be able to close his or her mouth in a physiologically relaxed position that easily. This is why the various techniques of relaxing the muscles and optimally maneuvering the jaws play such an important role in bite registration.

Without getting into technical details, a dentist can use physical therapy (massages, trigger point therapy), cold laser therapy, a TENS (transcutaneous electrical nerve stimulation) unit, or other avenues, to cause muscle relaxation in a patient before registering the optimal bite. Often, a dentist will take two different bites to correspond to the daytime and nighttime appliances.

REMOVABLE VERSUS FIXED ORTHOTIC APPLIANCES

Once a dentist records a patient's correct bite, he or she takes impressions (molds) of the patient's upper and lower teeth. At that point, the orthotic is ready to be fabricated by the dental laboratories.

The most common daytime appliance is a removable anatomic orthotic. A patient wears this orthotic, which mimics the anatomy of the chewing surface, over the lower teeth. The patient only removes this orthotic to brush his or her teeth and to sleep at night. A patient wears this type of orthotic for about twelve weeks, or until all TMD symptoms have alleviated.

The fixed orthotic is similar to the removable orthotic in function and anatomy, but it is bonded to the lower teeth and cannot be removed. When a dentist prescribes a fixed orthotic, the patient understands that at the end of therapy, he or she is going to require a full-mouth reconstruction with multiple crowns in order to make a permanent change to the bite.

Dentists make nighttime appliances for patients both to prevent grinding while sleeping and to address any airway obstruction issues.

TYPES OF TMD PATIENTS

There are, basically, four different sorts of patients who come through the doors of a dental practice:

- Patients who have painful symptoms of TMD.

- Patients who have compromised muscle functions due to TMD, but do not yet have the symptoms. These patients have limited mouth opening capabilities, or limited range of motion of the head and neck, but they have very little pain associated with the limitation.

- Patients who have self-destructive dentition. These patients have worn-down, fractured teeth, but they might have no pain associated with TMD.

- Patients who have TMD symptoms because of new occlusion established with orthodontics, full-mouth reconstructions, or dentures. These patients have not yet adapted to their new bite, or they need a bite adjustment.

CLICKING AND POPPING JOINTS: TO TREAT OR NOT TO TREAT

Some patients' jaws make a clicking or cracking sound in the joint when the jaws open or close, which is termed *crepitus*. Such a patient knows that his or her TMJ clicks and pops, and it has been clicking and popping, off and on, forever. This patient's question often is, "Does it need to be treated?" The consensus on that question is that although joint noise represents some abnormality, it does not always need to be treated. Altered disc morphology can cause clicking for many reasons, from subluxation (partial dislocation) of the joint due to osteoarthritis. A dentist makes the decision to treat joint sounds by considering the patient's pathology, symptoms, and age. If the function of the patient's joint is not compromised, and there is no pain or pathology associated with the joint, then the dentist will determine, most likely, that treatment is not needed.

The father of neuromuscular dentistry, Bernard Jacobson, famously said, "If it has been measured, it is a fact. If not, it is an opinion." That statement is the basis of neuromuscular dentistry, and it emphasizes why careful measurement is key to the neuromuscular approach.

CHAPTER THREE

SLEEP APNEA

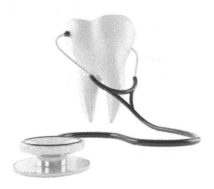

WE HEAR A GREAT DEAL ABOUT SLEEP APNEA TODAY; it is a growing global health issue, not just in developed countries, but also in developing countries. People often have a stereotyped view of the sleep apnea patient as an overweight, middle-aged man, but that is no longer accurate. Today, we see slim, young women and even children being diagnosed with sleep apnea. Increasing public awareness of this growing epidemic can lead to earlier screenings for the disease; these screenings can lead, in turn, to early diagnoses, better treatment options, and prevention of many related health issues.

Sleep apnea can be fatal; it can lead to many other chronic health conditions. If you have not had good sleep for even two days, you will feel fatigued and ready to collapse on the third day. Imagine not having adequate sleep for half your life and then going to work every day, trying to make the right decisions, driving to work, and taking care of your children in that state of sleep deprivation. There is biological evidence that sleep deprivation can actually impair some important physiological functions, like appetite and even regenerative responses. Your body needs rest; all your cells, which work constantly, need sleep to replicate and heal. The biggest impact of sleep deprivation is felt on the immune system. An impaired immune system leads to chronic diseases and other adverse health conditions.

Untreated sleep apnea increases the risk of having heart attacks by five, increases the risk of having strokes by two, and increases the risk of being in serious automobile accidents by five. Sleep apnea is related to premature death, diabetes, erectile dysfunction, hypertension, depression, obesity, and daytime fatigue.

SLEEP APNEA IN CHILDREN

Poor sleep among children can impact schoolwork; however, and more importantly, new research shows that poor sleep disrupts the secretion of the growth hormones, leading to stunted growth. In some cases, diagnosis and treatment of childhood sleep apnea has allowed a child to shoot up in height and gain weight suddenly.

New evidence points to the conclusion that many children who have been diagnosed with ADD and have been put on medications may actually be suffering from undiagnosed sleep apnea. Sleep deprivation can lead to crankiness, irritability, and inability to focus, all of which are symptoms commonly associated with ADD. Children diagnosed with ADD are often put on prescription medications, strong depressants that target the central nervous system and work to slow down a child.

SNORING AND SLEEP APNEA

Sleep-disordered breathing is described as sleep disturbances produced by normal breathing patterns. Snoring and sleep apnea are two of the most common sleep disorders that people have. *Snoring* is defined as breathing during sleep while producing harsh or sharp sounds, which are caused by the soft palate or uvula vibrating against the back of the throat or the base of the tongue. The vibration can be really loud or quite soft, but in either case it is a sign that the snoring person's breathing passage is partially blocked. This does not mean that every person who snores has sleep apnea; however, a person who snores should be screened for either apnea or hypopnea. Either of these disorders can lessen a person's oxygen intake to dangerously low levels and lead to some long-term chronic conditions.

Sleep apnea can cause headaches, fatigue, difficulty in conversation, and reduced work performance; it can also have a negative impact on relationships. I know couples who do not sleep together because of snoring problems.

WHAT IS SLEEP APNEA?

The word *apnea* means "without breath"; *apnea* is a cessation of breathing for at least ten seconds. There are several different types of sleep apnea, including *central sleep apnea* and obstructive sleep apnea. *Central sleep apnea* (CSA) is caused by the brain not telling the body to keep the throat and airway open while sleeping; in other words, it is a neurological issue. *Obstructive sleep apnea* (OSA) is a disorder in which breathing is briefly and repeatedly interrupted during sleep because of an obstruction in the airway. This periodic disruption and breathing causes an oxygen shortage to all parts of the body. Obstructive sleep apnea usually occurs when an individual's muscles in the back of the throat are not able to keep the throat open, despite that individual's efforts to breathe. This causes blockages in the airway and breathing interruption, or apnea, resulting in lowered blood oxygen levels.

Although we do not really know the exact connection between sleep apnea and heart disease, or between sleep apnea and other cardiovascular issues (such as high blood pressure, congestive heart failure, or heart attacks), we do see a link between them. People who develop these heart conditions frequently have sleep apnea.

Over time, an individual's lack of oxygen causes his or her blood vessels to narrow; eventually, the narrow blood vessels in the brain can obstruct blood flow into the brain and cause a stroke. In 2010, a study conducted at the National Institute of Health Studies found that OSA increases the risk of strokes in middle-aged and older men and women. Their study showed that even mild apnea can increase the risk of strokes in men, and this risk rises with the severity of the disease. Scientists continue to conduct research on sleep apnea's effects on so-called silent or mini strokes because evidence suggests that people are experiencing these brain-tissue-destroying episodes in their sleep due to apnea. Studies done by the National Stroke Association report that nearly two out of every three stroke survivors have sleep-disordered breathing, particularly OSA.

The Role of a Dentist in Screening for Sleep Apnea

Only 10 percent of individuals who suffer from sleep apnea have been diagnosed, and only one in every four of those diagnosed is being successfully treated. As a dentist, one of my biggest responsibilities is to screen patients for this potentially fatal condition and to see that my patients are referred to sleep clinics, if necessary, to make that diagnosis.

This diagnostic screening process starts with the practitioner taking the patient's vital signs, noting his or her body mass index (BMI), and recording his or her neck circumference. A few different circumferences of the neck indicate that a patient might have a closed or narrowed airway. For example, a man's 16.5-inch neck would indicate apnea, while a woman's neck that measured 15.5 inches or larger would indicate increased risk factors.

When a patient's BMI is greater than 30, he or she definitely has a big risk factor for obstructive sleep apnea. BMI is also the only reversible risk factor related to sleep apnea. If a patient lowers his or her BMI, he or she can decrease the risk of sleep apnea a great deal; obesity and sleep apnea are closely related to each other. Many people who have mild sleep apnea and are also overweight note that their apnea gets much better if they take steps to lose the extra pounds.

Dentists are most likely to see the visual signs associated with sleep apnea. The most common sign, for instance, is an enlarged tongue with tooth marks, or *scalloping*, on either side. An individual's large tongue can fall backwards during sleep and cause obstruction to his or her airway. Other markers of sleep apnea include the following: a large soft palate or uvula, a hypersensitive gag reflex, or enlarged tonsils. Too many dentists see these things but do not think to ask patients a simple question: "Do you snore?"

About 40 percent of the adult population suffers from some form of sleep disorder, ranging from mild snoring to serious OSA. Are you one of them? If so, your symptoms might include the following:

- Excessive daytime sleeping
- Loud, disruptive snoring
- Depression and irritability
- Sexual dysfunction
- Morning headaches
- Heart palpitations
- Memory loss and limited attention
- Grinding teeth at night

When a patient comes into my office, one of my colleagues or myself will give him or her a total health questionnaire, which includes questions on headaches, daytime sleepiness, and snoring. If the patient marks down that he or she is experiencing daytime sleepiness or snoring, a colleague or I will give him or her the Epworth Sleepiness scale questionnaire. This questionnaire is reproduced here:

SITUATION

(Refers to your usual way of life in recent times. Even if you have not done some of these things recently, try to work out how they would have affected you).

CHANCE OF DOZING

0 = would never doze

1 = slight chance of dozing

2 = moderate chance of dozing

3 = high chance of dozing

Sitting and reading	
Watching TV	
Sitting, inactive, in a public place	
Sitting as a passenger in a car for an hour	
Lying down in the afternoon	
Sitting and talking to someone	
Sitting quietly after a lunch without alcohol	
Sitting in a car, while stopped for a few minutes in traffic	
SCORE ANALYSIS TOTAL	

SCORE OF 1-3: You are getting enough sleep.

SCORE OF 4-8: You tend to be sleepy during the day; this is the average score.

SCORE OF 9-15: You are very sleepy and should seek medical advice.

SCORE OF 16 OR GREATER: You are dangerously sleepy and should seek medical advice.

Sleep bruxism, which is a dental condition, is also linked to sleep apnea. The latest evidence indicates that a patient with sleep apnea who also exhibits bruxism could be experiencing the latter as a physical protective mechanism against letting the jaw fall back during sleep. Via *bruxing*, or grinding, a patient could be trying to hold his or her teeth together so that the lower jaw does not slide backwards, thereby causing further obstruction of the airway.

Sleep bruxism is a different issue from regular clenching of the jaw; it is actually the third most common form of *parasomnia*, following snoring and obstructive sleep apnea. *Parasomnias* are categories of sleep disorders that involve abnormal and unnatural movement, similar to restless leg syndrome, which some people have before sleeping. These unnatural movements, behaviors, emotions, perceptions, or dreams occur while people are falling asleep, are sleeping, are between sleep stages, or are arising from sleep. Sleep bruxism happens to be one of the most common parasomnias. Because dentists often see it in conjunction with sleep apnea, noting the signs and symptoms of bruxism is an important part of dentists' screening process for sleep apnea.

Bruxism is a dental condition and is treated by a dentist. Sleep apnea, in contrast, may be screened by a dentist, but should be diagnosed only by a sleep physician.

If a dentist deems a patient at high risk for sleep apnea, based on the findings of the screening process, the dentist will then recommend the patient get a sleep study. These days, sleep studies can be done in a sleep laboratory or at a patient's home. The most important data collected from the sleep study is the AHI index. The AHI index, or the apnea-hypopnea index, is the measure of the severity of apnea in an individual. The AHI measures the number of times in an hour that a patient stops breathing. If there are five to fifteen events in an hour, the apnea is considered mild. If there are sixteen to thirty events in an hour, the apnea is considered moderate. If there are over thirty events an hour, the apnea is considered severe. The AHI index also reveals the duration of the cessations of breathing, along with the amount of oxygen desaturation in the blood.

A home sleep study should not be undertaken by children who are less than 14 years of age or in cases in which the patient has a neuromuscular disorder, like epilepsy, restless leg syndrome, or any kind of periodic limb movement. If the patient has severe congestive heart failure or a chronic obstructive pulmonary disease, like emphysema, and the dentist suspects sleep apnea, the dentist will send the patient directly to a sleep physician, since that patient's condition requires a hospital setting.

For children, the best way to do a screening for sleep apnea is through *acoustic pharyngometry* (measurement of the upper airways using reflective sound waves). Dentists use this assessment to measure the narrowest dimension in the upper airway. It is a simple, inexpensive test dentists can use to assess the risk of sleep apnea in children. A narrow airway may be inherited; children of parents who have sleep apnea are predisposed to sleep apnea.

TREATMENT OPTIONS

Options available to patients who want to solve their sleep disorders range from simple lifestyle changes to fairly invasive medical procedures. There are many contributing factors to snoring or sleep apnea that you can control. They include the following:

- Being overweight
- Smoking
- Drinking alcohol
- Using muscle relaxants or sleeping pills

All of these factors can affect the brain's control over the airway muscles during sleep.

The gold standard for treating severe sleep apnea is the CPAP. The CPAP is an air-pressure face mask that one uses while sleeping. It helps open up an individual's airway by providing positive pressure. An air pump connected to the mask constantly blows air through the air passageway at a level of pressure that does not allow the air passage to collapse. While the CPAP is very effective, many find it uncomfortable or even intolerable. If a patient cannot handle the CPAP, dentists often recommend an oral appliance, since such an appliance could reduce the severity of the sleep apnea, even if the results are less optimal compared to those of the CPAP.

Oral appliances are the most comfortable, least cumbersome treatment option for individuals suffering from mild to moderate sleep apnea. Two different kinds of oral appliances can be used for treating sleep apnea: the *mandibular advancement* (or repositioning) device and the tongue-retaining device. The mandibular advancement device moves the jaw, or mandible, forward, so that the tongue comes forward with it to help open the airway. Mandibular advancement devices are usually adjustable positioners. They may be simple devices, similar to teeth-whitening trays, which fit the upper and lower teeth and have a strap or a locking device between the two arches. There are many different names and brands of these devices available, but, essentially, they all do the same thing. Such a device holds the lower jaw forward while the patient sleeps so that the jaw and the tongue do not fall back and cause an obstruction to the airway. The FDA has approved these devices. Tongue-retaining devices, which are intended to hold the tongue forward and out of the way of the airway, are not used as much, and they are not FDA-approved.

The last-resort option for obstructive sleep apnea is surgery. The American Academy of Sleep Medicine currently endorses only one type of surgery: *uvulopalatopharyngoplasty* (UPPP), which is a surgical procedure in which the surgeon tries to reshape the patient's palate or uvula. The extensiveness of the surgery depends on what tissues are blocking the airway; the surgery might even include a tonsillectomy if enlarged tonsils have caused the obstruction. Surgical procedures may not be helpful in every patient, and their long-term effectiveness is not proven. In fact, the UPPP has a short-term success rate of only 50 percent, which is not very high. The success rate of an oral appliance is comparable to or better than the surgical option. That is why dentists use less-invasive options, like the CPAP and use oral appliances, as the first line of treatment.

ADVANTAGES OF ORAL APPLIANCES

The advantages of oral appliances over surgery or CPAP include the following: they are inexpensive; they are non-invasive, compared to surgery; they are easy to fabricate; they are versatile; they are easy for traveling; they are very portable, small, and comfortable; and they also have a high rate of compliance. Patients actually use them, as opposed to the CPAP. One study indicated that the usual wear time for CPAP is 4.5 hours in a 24-hour period. A person sleeps an average of 8 to 9 hours; therefore, this means that 50 percent of the time that patient who has sleep apnea tries sleeping with a closed-up airway because he or she is not able to wear the CPAP for more than 4.5 hours. Some people wake up often because the mask is uncomfortable; they have more frequent disturbances during the night, which leads to sleep fragmentation.

LIMITATIONS OF ORAL APPLIANCES

One disadvantage of oral appliances is that sometimes they can be uncomfortable for patients during initial use because they can cause some soreness of teeth and gums. In some cases when first inserting the appliance, a patient can have extreme dry mouth or its opposite, excessive salivation. The appliance can put pressure on the teeth and change the position of the teeth if those teeth are already mobile, especially if other periodontal issues are present.

Patients can experience some temporomandibular joint discomfort, too, which is why it is so important for dentists to screen patients for TMD. Whenever a dentist gives a patient an oral appliance, it is very important for the dentist to see the patient again after the first two or three weeks. This is a period of adaptation. There will be some soreness, and some adjustments required. Once the patient is comfortable with wearing the appliance and all adjustments have been fine-tuned, the dentist will recommend the patient have a home sleep study in order to see if his or her AHI has dropped down to acceptable levels and if his or her oxygen saturation level is good. Sleep technicians and physicians conduct and supervise the final test of the appliance: an overnight sleep study. Oral appliance delivery and follow-up is a process made up of plenty of checks and balances, so a dentist can make sure that when he or she delivers an oral appliance to a patient that the appliance is effective and is doing what it is supposed to do. After that, the dentist sees that patient yearly in order to be sure that everything is still working and in its proper place.

GOOD CANDIDATES FOR
ORAL APPLIANCES

For a dentist, the most important element of assessing a patient is probably determining the lack of periodontal disease in that patient, since an oral appliance does put pressure on the teeth. A dentist will try to get the patient's gum disease under control first. It is also important that the patient has no significant temporomandibular joint (TMJ) problems and is at a normal weight or only moderately overweight. If the patient's apnea is being caused by a weight problem, the dentist will want to try to get the patient to lose the weight.

In the case of a patient who has sleep apnea and presents an underdeveloped lower jaw, one of the likely reasons for his or her apnea is that the lower jaw is falling back; in that case, a dentist will know that bringing the lower jaw forward is going to help. If the airway obstruction is behind the tongue, that is important for the dentist to know, too. The dentist needs to know that the apnea is being caused because of the tongue position, not because of a nasal problem. If a patient has a deviated septum, rhinitis, some kind of nasal polyp, or any kind of obstruction in the nose, a dentist will not be able to help that patient with an oral appliance.

A certain set of oral appliances has an extension going up under the lip that puts pressure on the nose from inside the mouth and keeps the nostrils dilated. Using such an appliance can help a patient if he or she has a minor issue with nasal obstruction. A dentist will refer patients who have major issues, like a deviated septum or nasal polyps, to an ENT specialist.

Mild to moderate sleep apnea patients are the best candidates for the appliance approach; severe sleep apnea really does require a CPAP. That said, if a patient has moderate to severe sleep apnea but cannot tolerate a CPAP, then of course a dentist will strongly recommend oral appliances. This recommendation is also true for patients who do not respond to weight loss programs or changes in sleep position. It is also for those who refuse surgical treatment, or for those who have already had surgical corrections of nasal and throat obstructions that did not solve their OSA completely. In those cases, repositioning the jaw is the next best thing to getting rid of an obstruction behind the tongue.

HORMONAL CHANGES RELATED TO SLEEP APNEA

Leptin is a hormone that suppresses appetite and promotes weight loss. When people sleep, their levels of *leptin* are elevated, even during daytime sleep. When people have problems sleeping, their leptin levels are lowered as much as 19 percent. When people have lowered leptin levels, they will feel hungry when they get up, and they will experience weight gain. Low leptin levels may be a primary cause of obesity for people who have sleep apnea.

Ghrelin, a peptide produced in the stomach and hypothalamus, is the only known appetite-stimulating hormone in a human being. Usually, people's ghrelin levels tend to rise before meals and decrease after meals. People who do not sleep well will experience an increase in ghrelin levels and hunger; in particular, these people will crave calorie-dense carbohydrates. Even a single night of sleep deprivation is enough to raise ghrelin levels and make an individual hungry the next day.

Insulin is a hormone produced by the pancreas. High insulin levels in the body cause fat storage. Insulin resistance is one of the key components of metabolic syndrome and, of course, diabetes. When an individual has decreased insulin sensitivity and decreased glucose effectiveness, his or her insulin resistance is increased; this is what happens to people with OSA. Treatment of OSA actually improves a patient's glucose metabolism. Treatment can help with diabetes by aiding in the maintenance of the insulin and blood sugar levels.

Cortisol, or *hydrocortisone,* is a *glucocorticoid* produced by the adrenal glands and released in response to stress and the levels of blood glucocorticoids. Sleep deprivation makes a person's body think that it is stressed, which prompts the body to increase cortisol levels. This is not an overnight effect; it takes about three weeks of sleep deprivation to change the levels of cortisol in the body. However, cortisol increases the body's level of blood sugar and can play an adverse role in patients who are diabetics.

The growth hormone stimulates growth, cell reproduction, and regeneration, and which is secreted during stage-III sleep. If it is reduced, it has an adverse effect on an individual's growth and development, especially if it is reduced in a child.

Prolactin is a hormone produced by the pituitary gland. It has a major role in lactation, and it is also a significant regulator of the immune system. If an individual's prolactin is low, his or her immunity decreases. Low prolactin also increases an individual's carbohydrate cravings because of elevated insulin.

As you can see, many different hormones have connections to conditions like obesity, diabetes, and lowered immune systems. Oral appliances can reduce sleep fragmentation, improve oxygen saturation, and increase stage III sleep. These benefits, in turn, increase leptin and appetite suppression, decrease ghrelin and appetite stimulation, improve glucose tolerance, and reduce cortisol and the stress response. A dentist plays a significant role in affecting a patient's overall health by helping that patient manage his or her sleep apnea. Dental sleep medicine can play a vital role in managing the obesity epidemic.

CHAPTER FOUR

Patient FAQs

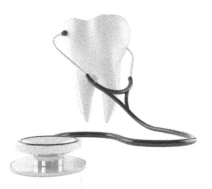

Why Can't I Just Get a Regular Cleaning Along with My Exam?

A dentist or a dental hygienist performs cleaning of a patient's teeth and gums as treatment. This cleaning may be a preventative treatment to avert gingivitis, or it may be a therapeutic treatment performed on a patient who already has gum disease.

When a patient comes in to a dental office, the dentist or hygienist will perform a comprehensive examination on that patient in order to arrive at a specific, individual treatment plan. The treatment plan is based on a diagnosis made after a thorough examination performed using all the available diagnostic aids. When a dentist looks at the patient's gums, he or she notes the gums' color, shape, and size. The dentist records areas of the patient's mouth that bleed on probing, pocket depth, and gum recession. Based on a determination of whether the patient's gums are healthy or unhealthy, the dentist will classify the cleanings as either preventative or therapeutic.

Preventative cleaning is what most patients think of as regular cleaning. Every dentist does preventative cleaning differently. At my office, for instance, when a patient comes in for his or her first visit, my colleagues and I look at everything related to the patient's teeth, including the jaws, the head, and the neck. After that, we make a diagnosis. Once we have made a diagnosis of the patient's gums and their health, we make a treatment plan. Before that, my colleagues and I do not know the kind of cleaning the patient needs. After that, the patient comes back for another visit to get his or her cleaning. The dental cleaning is part of his treatment, not part of his exam. At my office, we make that separation because we want patients to understand that cleaning is not just polishing teeth to make them look brighter or whiter. A dental cleaning is meant to keep teeth and gums healthy. Before making an appointment for a patient's dental cleaning, my colleagues and I want to know how much time to allocate to that appointment. We need to see how much *calculus* (calcified buildup on teeth) or *plaque* (non-calcified buildup on teeth) the patient has. We need to see if there is a need to anesthetize or not, or if the cleaning is going to be a quick procedure because the patient's oral hygiene is excellent. We would like to determine if the patient requires detailed instructions on brushing, flossing, and so forth in order to improve his or her oral hygiene. A dental cleaning appointment based on all this information can take anywhere from 30 minutes to two and a half hours. That is why a patient does not get his or her cleaning along with an exam, at least in our office.

In addition, it is important to remember that 80 percent of the adult American population has periodontal disease. A patient has to belong to the 20 percent with no gum disease in order to get a regular cleaning only. If you have not had a dental cleaning once every six months, your expectation of "just needing a regular cleaning" must change.

ASIDE FROM WHAT YOU SEE, HOW DO YOU DIAGNOSE THE HEALTH OF MY GUMS?

To get an accurate assessment of a patient's *gingival*, or gum, health, my colleagues and I rely on several tests. One is the BANA test. In this test, we scrape out a bit of tartar from one of the deepest pockets in the mouth, smear it on a strip, and put it in a machine that relays a color code (like a litmus test). The strip changes color depending on whether the patient has the specific bacteria that cause periodontal disease. Some people have these bacteria, and some people do not. People who do not have the bacteria are not predisposed to periodontal disease. The BANA test does not quantify the level of bacteria present in a person's mouth, and it is not specific to the exact species of bacteria causing the disease. An oral DNA test, in contrast, is very specific. We do this test by having a patient swish with a solution and spit the solution and saliva into a test tube. We then send the saliva sample to a laboratory to be analyzed.

We can conduct two different oral DNA tests to find periodontal disease. The first test identifies the specific bacteria and determines if it is a high, low, or moderate risk in terms of causing periodontal disease. The test also identifies if the bacteria's level is above the threshold that can cause infection in the patient's mouth.

The second test is genetic and looks for the presence or absence of the Interleukin-1 (IL-1) gene in a patient's DNA. If the gene is present, the patient has a higher risk of getting periodontal disease. In addition, the patient will have a tendency to get other chronic inflammatory diseases, including rheumatoid arthritis and cardiovascular disease. This test can be used on children who show early signs of periodontal disease or have a family history of it. When a child receives early screening for the presence or absence of the IL-1 gene, his or her parent can make certain changes in the child's diet, lifestyle, and oral hygiene practices. These changes, if made early enough, can prevent the clinical manifestations of many diseases.

DEPENDING ON WHAT YOU FIND, WHAT ARE THE DIFFERENT TYPES OF CLEANING YOU MIGHT USE?

Basic dental cleaning, or *dental prophylaxis*, is a preventative treatment used to keep the gums in a healthy condition. It involves removal of plaque, removal of stains above the gum line, and polishing of teeth.

When a patient has so much build-up of plaque or stains that even a visual examination of the teeth is impossible for a dentist, then that patient needs a thorough cleaning, or a *full-mouth debridement*. A full-mouth debridement can be categorized as a diagnostic cleaning, because a dentist reexamines the patient's teeth and gums after such a cleaning to arrive at a final diagnosis.

The third kind of cleaning is *scaling and root planning*, also known as *deep cleaning* in layman's terms. During this cleaning, the hygienist or dentist uses ultrasonic scalars or hand scalars to scale the teeth, remove all the calcified plaque (above and below the gums), and, if necessary, plane the roots of the teeth to get rid of tartar and make the root surface smooth.

To control the bacteria that cause gum infections, dentists can use many adjunctive therapies. Dentists can use antibacterial solutions to wash out the depths of the pockets in the mouth. In addition, dentists can place local antimicrobial agents or antibiotics in the base of the pockets. These antibiotics are slow, sustained-release medications that can stay in the pockets for almost ten days. Dentists may also use LDR, a pulsated low-level laser, to lower bacterial risk or bacterial count in the deep parts of the pockets that cannot be reached with other dental instruments.

The most important part of periodontal therapy is patients' frequent return visits for *periodontal maintenance*, which should occur every three to four months. Periodontal maintenance is the type of cleaning done after scaling and root planning to manage the disease and slow down its progression. A patient may assume, "Well, I got a scaling and root cleaning, and now I can come every six months," or "I can just get a regular cleaning after this treatment." Unfortunately, periodontal disease, like diabetes or hypertension, is a disease that has no permanent cure. It can be controlled only by periodic, timely treatments every three to four months. Studies show that the pathogenic bacteria that cause periodontal disease reach a level that can cause disease in about 9 to 12 weeks after a cleaning. The purpose of bringing patients in after a shorter amount of time, three to four months, is to prevent a patient's bacterial load from rising above threshold and causing reinfection.

WHAT IS TOOTH DECAY?

Tooth decay, or *dental caries*, is a transmissible bacterial infection. A *cavity* on a tooth is just a symptom of that bacterial infection. The clinical treatment of this infection is still largely based on the restorative model of dentistry; however, just putting in fillings does not halt the process of the disease. That is why most preventative-thinking dentists who like to do minimally invasive dentistry or perform the most conservative form of dentistry believe in CAMBRA (Caries Management by Risk Assessment).

Dentists believe that two different types of bacteria cause tooth decay: *streptococci* and *lactobacillus*. These bacteria generate acid from the carbohydrates people eat, and that acid is what breaks down the outer layer of the tooth, called *enamel*. After a certain amount of damage to the enamel occurs, a process known as *demineralization*, a cavitation or cavity formation becomes visible on the surface of the tooth. The amount of bacteria in the mouth is directly proportional to the number of cavities a person is likely to get. Having adequate saliva is probably the most important factor in cavity prevention. The saliva provides a buffer and extra calcium and phosphate that can reverse the early damage caused by demineralization. Saliva can neutralize the acid that comes from the bacteria. It allows the calcium and phosphate to go back into the enamel, which is a process called *remineralization.*

According to CAMBRA, a patient will continue developing tooth decay, if there is an imbalance in his or her oral environment, or some sort of disharmony between the protective factors and the destructive factors in the mouth. This causes more demineralization than remineralization. The former is the ultimate cause of tooth decay.

The factors that cause more demineralization in the mouth are the presence of these bacteria, poor salivation, poor dietary habits, and poor oral hygiene habits. The protective factors include the following: producing an adequate amount of healthy saliva; using more products that contain baking soda or anything that neutralizes acids; using sealants or anti-microbial agents, like xylitol, chlorhexidine, or topical fluoride; using other remineralization products; maintaining a good diet and good oral hygiene; decreasing the frequency of snacking; and increasing the levels of calcium and phosphate in the saliva.

A cavity, or the caries lesion, is a symptom of the caries disease. The real causes of the tooth damage are bacterial infection, poor dietary habits, and *xerostomia*, which is dry mouth or lack of saliva. Treatment should focus on treating the disease, not just repairing the symptoms by restoring the tooth. That is why CAMBRA focuses on detection and treatment of both the cavitated and non-cavitated lesions of the mouth. When examining patients, CAMBRA practitioners look at the reasons for any imbalance between the protective and destructive factors in the mouth.

A dentist can do salivary flow tests on a patient to find out if he or she has inadequate saliva. The dentist checks the saliva for the presence and count of a certain bacteria called *streptococcus mutans*. The baseline saliva test measures the stimulated flow rate and the level of pathogenic bacteria.

Then the dentist can use a risk assessment form specific to tooth decay for evaluating the pathogenic or negative factors versus the protective factors in the patient's mouth. Dentists may use one of two different forms based on the patient's age. Dentists use one form for patients who are zero to six years of age, and they use the other form for patients who are six years of age and older. This is because there is a difference in the kinds of oral hygiene practiced by children and adults.

If a dentist fills a cavity without addressing its cause, there is a high probability that tooth decay will occur around that filling and that filling will have to be replaced; eventually, the patient might need a bigger, more extensive restoration or a crown.

During exams, dentists see both cavitated and non-cavitated lesions. When a tooth's enamel starts getting affected by the acid, the lesions produced by that acid go through different stages before becoming clinically significant defects (the point at which one needs to restore them). Non-cavitated caries, in the form of white and brown spots, are reversible lesions that dentists can arrest by chemical or mechanical means. There are different ways of addressing a cavity before a dentist needs to pick up a *handpiece* (or dentist's drill) and physically take out carious tooth structure and fill it. That is why dentists need to be looking at the dental caries process from a preventative standpoint rather than a restorative standpoint. Our office, for instance, is geared toward minimally invasive dentistry. My colleagues and I do not like to remove tooth structure and like to conserve tooth structure as much as possible.

WHAT DO YOU MEAN BY "MINIMALLY INVASIVE," AND WHAT IS MINIMALLY INVASIVE TECHNOLOGY?

The essence of minimally invasive dentistry is to be able to diagnose a cavity before it becomes a cavity, or to diagnose gum disease before it has caused irreversible destruction to the tissues supporting the teeth. At our office, for example, we use diagnostic imaging and digital radiography, which give us instant, enhanced images of patients' mouths with minimal radiation and without using toxic chemicals. We conduct noninvasive caries detection by using lasers, magnification, and intraoral cameras, and by doing tooth decay screening and management. We use patient questionnaires to assess patients' habits, diets, and so forth. For instance, we use the saliva test for bacteria, which helps control the disease in a minimally invasive manner. We also conduct oral cancer detection by using something called a VELscope; doing so potentially saves lives by locating precancerous lesions in their earliest stages. That is minimally invasive.

Much of our minimally invasive technology comes at the diagnostic stage.

We also use it in treatment, such as using a laser or air abrasion to remove tooth structure rather than a drill. If a patient is allergic to tetracycline or does not want to have any antibiotics placed in his or her mouth, then a colleague or I can use a pulsated laser to reduce bacterial count; this also allows treatment without any systemic effects. These lasers can stimulate cell growth and regeneration, reduce bleeding, and provide anti-inflammatory and bio-stimulating effects.

CAD/CAM technology (Computer Aided Design/ Computer Aided Manufacturing) allows dentists to do same-day, indirect restorations on patients without having to send an impression of a patient's mouth to a laboratory and wait for a crown or an inlay to be fabricated and sent back two to three weeks later. Now, dentists can prepare the tooth and permanently cement the crown on the same day. As a result, the patient no longer has to wait for a few weeks wearing a temporary crown, which might fit poorly or leak. When a patient's missing tooth needs to be replaced, dentists can suggest an implant as a less invasive choice, since installing an implant does not involve cutting the teeth on either side of the space as is needed while doing a bridge.

WHY TREAT BABY TEETH? THEY ARE JUST GOING TO FALL OUT ANYWAY.

Contrary to what many parents think, baby teeth are very important. They definitely should not be taken out or left to decay just because the child is going to have another set of teeth later on. These teeth need to be saved until the root of the permanent tooth underneath each one is formed enough, ready to erupt, and ready to come out.

However, there are certain times when a dentist does need to take a patient's baby teeth out. Usually, when a child has a cavity on one of his or her baby teeth, the dentist would want to restore it. In some instances, a patient may be have missing permanent teeth; if so, the dentist will want to conserve the baby tooth until the patient is ready to restore the space with a more permanent solution, like an implant or a bridge.

A recent study investigated how pain in the mouth due to cavities in children is affecting children's school performance. Infection and cavities in young patients' baby teeth should be addressed because they are painful for a child and because they affect the permanent teeth, too.

Healthy baby teeth are necessary for chewing and for getting good nutrition. Much of people's absorption and digestion of food starts in the mouth. In addition, people learn to speak as children. The tongue rests in certain spots behind the teeth in order for people to enunciate and pronounce certain words. If those teeth are missing, an individual will not experience proper speech development. The present baby teeth stimulate jawbone development. If the teeth are not there and the function of chewing does not occur, then jaw development is hindered.

In addition, society requires people have healthy teeth in order to smile and present an attractive appearance. Children can suffer self-esteem issues or be bullied when they have missing front teeth. One of the most important functions of baby teeth is that they hold spaces for permanent teeth. They reserve space for permanent teeth and guide those teeth into position.

Losing one tooth will make other teeth shift to that tooth's space; suddenly, the permanent tooth will not have any space to erupt in the right place. This causes other issues, such as crowding and impaction of permanent teeth.

WHAT CAN PARENTS DO TO PREVENT TOOTH DECAY?

Dentists hear this all the time: "My children brush two times a day, but every time I take them to the dentist, they still have cavities." As I wrote earlier, dental caries, or tooth decay, is caused by transmissible bacterial infection; if a parent has a high incidence of caries, his or her child will too. If a parent puts something in his or her mouth and then puts it in his or her child's mouth, the parent is transferring caries-causing bacteria. Not many parents understand that they must care for their own teeth to keep their children's teeth healthy. In addition, when children eat sugary, starchy, or sticky foods that feed bacteria, and their teeth are not cleaned regularly, the bacteria will help produce acid and cause decay to the teeth. Parents must encourage their children to develop healthy oral hygiene habits, like brushing and flossing after every meal; parents must also encourage their children to reduce their intake of sugary snacks, sodas, and juices.

An untreated tooth can cause an abscess. The infection can go down to the permanent tooth bud while that bud is still developing. This can cause a malformed or underdeveloped permanent tooth.

Until children are eight years old, parents should be brushing their children's teeth. These young children do not know how to brush. Moreover, they cannot brush effectively because they do not have the kind of dexterity needed to clean their teeth well. Their teeth should be brushed in the morning and right before bed with fluoridated toothpaste. Parents should limit the amount of fruit juice, sweet drinks, and snacks their children consume, and they should never put their children to bed or down for a nap with a bottle or Sippy cup containing milk or fruit juice. The bottle or Sippy cup should only have water in it. If you must give the child juice, dilute it with water.

Never dip a pacifier in sugar or honey. If you do have to give a pacifier to your child, make sure there is nothing sugary in his or her mouth for long periods of time before or after giving the pacifier, since sugar gets broken down into acid by bacteria. Snacks like cheese, yogurt, fruits, and vegetables are better for children than chips, crackers, and other foods that contain carbohydrates.

Start regular dental visits when a child turns one year old. When you take your children to a dental provider, get them fluoride treatments, get them dental sealants, and get their saliva checked. Find out if your children have a risk for cavities, and address it right then. It is easier to address that topic when a patient is two than it is when he or she is fourteen. It is easier to create better oral hygiene habits when children are five or six years old than it is when they are teenagers. By that time, most of the damage has already occurred.

Your one-year-old's first dental visit is a well-baby check-up. At this check-up, the dentist should go over proper brushing and oral hygiene. He or she will evaluate potentially bad habits, like sucking the thumb and biting the lip, that need to be stopped by a certain age. The dentist will look at other issues, too; for example, if the teeth shown in the X-ray are bigger than what the jaw growth is likely to accommodate later on, the dentist will evaluate potential crowding down the road.

A child under the age of eight or nine should not take tetracyclines or a high amount of fluoride in water because doing so affects the development of the enamel in the tooth. A child's baby teeth are going to last five to ten years, or even longer, so parents and children should take care of these baby teeth.

MY DENTIST SAYS I NEED TO TAKE OUT MY WISDOM TEETH, BUT THEY'RE NOT BOTHERING ME. DO I REALLY NEED TO HAVE THEM REMOVED?

Wisdom teeth need not be removed if they are healthy, have grown in completely, are positioned correctly, and are biting properly with the opposite teeth. Most of the time, wisdom teeth have no space to grow in properly. Sometimes they emerge only partially through the gums, sometimes they grow at different angles in the jaw, and sometimes they become impacted or trapped within the jaw. The American Dental Association recommends a wisdom tooth should be removed if that wisdom tooth has partially emerged through the gums because this partial emergence increases the chance of the bacterial infection *pericoronitis*. That means that there is a flap behind or on top of the wisdom tooth because the tooth has not been able to come out all the way. Bacteria and food can get caught under that flap, which causes an infection.

Un-erupted wisdom teeth, which are expected to grow in crookedly and damage other teeth, should be removed. It is important to get the wisdom tooth out before that happens. If a fluid-filled sac or cyst develops around the un-erupted wisdom tooth that can damage the surrounding tissue or bone, then it needs to be removed. If there are deep pockets around the wisdom teeth, and if the patient cannot floss or brush the area effectively, then bacteria may harbor around the wisdom teeth, causing yet another infection.

WHAT ARE THE RISKS ASSOCIATED WITH REMOVING WISDOM TEETH?

There are some risks associated with removing wisdom teeth. For instance, there is a risk of fracture, numbness, and nerve damage. The removal may not be a minor surgery. If the reasons to remove the wisdom teeth are not there, a dentist will not recommend their removal. The risks of removal depend on the following: the type of impaction of the wisdom teeth (in other words, how hard it is going to be to get the teeth out); the age of the patient (a younger patient will heal faster and have less post-operative discomfort); and any underlying medical issues a patient may have.

Do I Need to Floss My Teeth if I Brush Two Times a Day and After Every Meal?

Flossing helps remove the plaque that has built up between the teeth and around the gum line. It removes bacteria that can cause cavities between teeth. To maintain healthy gums and healthy teeth, especially between the teeth, people need to floss. Toothbrush bristles do not reach between teeth. No matter how much a person brushes his or her teeth, he or she cannot clean a tight contact between two teeth effectively, which is why flossing is necessary. Water picks work well to mechanically wash away plaque from embrasures (triangular spaces between the teeth above and below the area of contact), but flossing is still required in order to reach contact areas.

There are many ways to floss. The most common method is still that of using the traditional floss thread. There are various other products in the market, such as interproximal brushes, toothpicks, floss holders, and water flossers, which are oral irrigators or dental water jets. However, traditional dental floss is still considered the most effective product. Whatever you choose to use, remember that flossing is important. That is why dentists use the saying, "Floss the teeth you want to keep."

What Kind of a Toothbrush Should I Get? Do I Really Need to Get an Expensive Electric Toothbrush or is a Manual Toothbrush Okay?

A manual toothbrush works well. An extra-soft or soft bristle brush is recommended. Combining a hard bristle brush and some abrasive toothpaste can cause excessive wear to the teeth and gums, and it might even damage the tissues. Using the full twenty strokes on each side to brush, along with the right angulation and technique, is more important than the kind of toothbrush used. A dental hygienist will be happy to show the proper technique.

For people who have a tendency to press too hard when they brush, using an electric toothbrush is a good idea. Electric toothbrushes will stop when too much pressure is applied to the bristles.

Dentists also recommend electric toothbrushes for patients who have gingivitis and periodontitis, as well as for patients who lack the manual dexterity to brush with the right technique. For a patient who has a healthy mouth with no issues and little plaque or build-up, a manual toothbrush will do just fine.

HOW OFTEN SHOULD
TOOTHBRUSHES BE CHANGED?

Toothbrushes need to be changed every three months, or earlier if the bristles get splayed and loose their shape. The other time you should change your toothbrush comes when you have had a strep infection or have been sick.

Toothbrushes should never be shared, especially with children. Fluoridated toothpaste is not recommended for children under five years as they may ingest it. A pea-sized amount of toothpaste is all that is necessary to brush your teeth.

ARE MOUTHWASHES NECESSARY
OR EFFECTIVE?

Mouthwashes are never a substitute for brushing or flossing. They are good mouth fresheners. Medicated mouthwashes or anti-bacterial rinses are usually dispensed by a dentist's prescription and should be used per the dentist's instructions. Over-the-counter mouthwashes should be used with discretion and discussed with your dentist.

WHY IS MY DENTIST RECOMMENDING A CROWN INSTEAD OF A FILLING?

A crown is a tooth-shaped cap placed over a tooth. A dentist uses a crown on a patient to restore a tooth's shape, size, and strength, or to improve its appearance. When the dentist cements the crown in place, that crown covers the entire visible portion of the tooth that is above the gum line. A crown protects a weak tooth from breaking and helps hold together a cracked tooth. When a tooth is treated with a root canal, it lacks blood supply and becomes brittle and prone to fracture.

Stress-bearing teeth that have had root canals should be crowned for protection. A dentist will also recommend crowns for instances when a patient complains of symptoms that sound like cracked tooth syndrome. These symptoms usually include pain when chewing and temperature sensitivity.

In addition, a dentist will want to put a crown on a tooth to restore what is already broken, or to preserve a tooth if part of it has been worn down from grinding. If a tooth has lost most of its enamel, a dentist will recommend a crown to restore the tooth's original shape, form, and function. A dentist will also put a crown on a tooth that needs or has a very large filling if the tooth structure around the filling is fragile or insufficient for adequate support of the filling.

If a tooth has erupted in a misshapen state, has become severely discolored, or has some intrinsic stain that cannot be bleached, a dentist will put a crown on that tooth to protect it and improve its appearance. Dentists also use crowns over implants to replace missing teeth.

Many people ask what the difference is between metal, porcelain, resin, and gold crowns. Gold is a good material for crowns, and it wears in the mouth like natural tooth structure does. Gold is very forgiving when a patient is a bruxer and grinds and clenches his or her teeth. It lasts for a long time and is biologically compatible. It does not rust and it does not corrode. These days, for aesthetic reasons, most people want tooth-colored crowns, which is why porcelain is used to make crowns more often than metal. Dentists bond the porcelain to metal to combine the strength of the metal and the aesthetics of porcelain. In porcelain-to-metal crowns, the metal used maybe high-noble metal, which contains gold, platinum, or palladium. It may also be a base metal, which contains nickel chromium or cobalt. Base metals can sometimes cause allergies, and they may not be as biocompatible as high noble metals are.

The porcelain that bonds to a metal can sometimes chip away from that metal. When that happens, the porcelain cannot be bonded back to the metal. A dentist can try to repair it with other materials, but the resulting bond is weaker.

The metal under the porcelain can sometimes cause discoloration along the crown's gum line. This can be a problem around the front teeth, where aesthetics is a major concern. Today, there are completely metal-free materials available for fabricating crowns, and these materials do not pose the above-mentioned problems. Some of these materials are similar in strength to porcelain-and-metal crowns, if not stronger.

These days, different dental materials come into the market constantly, each boasting superior strength, better biocompatibility, and increased durability. Dentists perform dentistry on patients over their lifetimes using materials that are more prevalent and popular during those periods of time. Over time, a patient may end up with many different materials in his or her mouth. One patient could have silver fillings on one tooth, a white filling on the other, and maybe a gold crown on a back tooth and a porcelain crown in the front. All of these materials have different rates of wear and different life expectancies. That does not mean a dentist needs to take everything out and try to make all the materials in one patient's mouth the same. However, there are certain disadvantages to having dissimilar materials in a single mouth.

All-porcelain crowns are suitable for patients who have metal allergies, but some of these crowns tend to wear on the opposing teeth more because they are even harder than natural tooth structure is. In the cases of people who grind or clench their teeth, it is important for dentists to address these parafunctional habits first, before restoring any teeth with crowns.

WHY IS MY DENTIST SAYING I NEED A ROOT CANAL? I ALREADY HAD A FILLING (OR CROWN).

A tooth's nerve can become irritated, inflamed, and infected due to deep decay near the pulp or involving the pulp, repeated dental procedures on a tooth (that is, mechanical trauma), a crack on the tooth, trauma to the face, or a large and/or deep filling placed near the pulp.

When caries reach the inner chamber of a tooth and involve the pulp or nerve of the tooth, bacteria start multiplying within the pulp chamber and cause an infection there. This, in turn, can cause an abscess or a pus-filled sac to develop at the end of the tooth's root. This abscess can spread and cause a swelling in other areas of the face, neck, or head. It can also cause bone loss around the root and drainage through the gums or cheek to the outer skin.

When a dentist conducts a root canal, he or she removes the pulp, bacteria, decayed nerve tissue, and related debris from the tooth. The dentist accomplishes this process by using root canal files. After the dentist has thoroughly cleaned the root, he or she shapes, enlarges, irrigates (using anti-microbial solutions), dries, and seals (with inert materials) the tooth. Root canals have a success rate of more then 95 percent. A dentist performs a root canal on a patient in order to help him or her retain his or her own, natural tooth. The only other way of getting rid of a tooth infection is through extraction.

SIGNS OF NEEDING A ROOT CANAL

- Severe toothache upon chewing or applying pressure to the tooth.
- Prolonged sensitivity or pain to hot and cold temperatures even after the stimulus is removed.
- Discoloration or darkening of the tooth, which indicates a dying nerve and is seen most commonly after trauma to the tooth.
- Swelling and tenderness in the gums or a persistent or recurring draining abscess on the gums.
- The tooth throbs for no reason, gets worse upon lying down, and wakes the individual up at night.

Today, endodontists have techniques, materials, and machines that can often perform this procedure in a single visit; what's more, the procedure is totally painless. If you last had a root canal ten years ago, you may be surprised to find there is a huge difference between that and the experience today. Root canals are not anything to fear, and they are definitely not painful. What is painful is when someone lets a tooth get infected to the extent that even a local anesthetic does not numb it easily. At that point, any procedure would be painful. It is important to prevent this from happening and get care sooner rather than late. Tooth infections do not resolve themselves. They do not get completely resolved even with antibiotics. A dentist must treat a patient's infected tooth in order to get rid of the infection.

Never be afraid to ask your dentist a question about any issue relating to your health or treatment. Fortunately, with today's evidence-based dentistry, visual technology allows each patient to see and understand what the dentist is seeing. That allows the dentist and patient to come to a *co-diagnosis*, a process in which the dentist and patient come to a conclusion as a team after interpreting the various results of the test(s) done together, so there is no doubt or question about the recommended treatment plan. That is the ideal relationship between the dentist and the patient – one in which questions are asked and answered freely, and one in which trust is retained from the first visit through the ongoing treatment. The patient's trust in the dentist is validated by evidence every step of the way. This is why dentists preform evidence based dentistry: so that each patient can do what is best for him or her, with no doubts about what is necessary and why.

CHAPTER FIVE

NUTRITION AND DENTISTRY

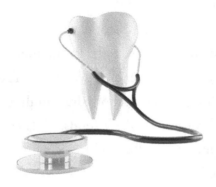

NUTRITION PLAYS A VERY IMPORTANT ROLE IN DENTISTRY because the pathogenesis of dental caries, or tooth decay, is based on diet and bacteria. If there is no food in the mouth, then there are no carbohydrates or sugars that can be broken down into acids by the bacteria present in the mouth. Then, there would be no cavities on teeth. As you can see, what people take into their mouths is very important to the way cavities occur

Besides that, of course, nutrition is important for the entire body. This works both ways. If there are not any teeth, or if there is disease in the mouth and a person cannot eat properly, or if food cannot be digested because chewing is not done properly, then the nutrition of the entire body is affected. When the body is malnourished, the oral cavity or the mouth shows the malnourishment very quickly and obviously through various different symptoms and signs. This happens because the oral cavity is so sensitive. The cells lining the mouth, unlike those in the skin, get replaced every few days instead of every few weeks or months. Any kind of deficiency in the diet that affects the cell replication of the mucous membrane or the inner lining of the mouth will show up quickly as red, swollen, or ulcerated mucous membrane.

Over 2,000 years ago, Aristotle wrote that he saw sweet figs would produce damage to the teeth. In the nineteenth century and twentieth century, people experienced a huge increase in dental decay because of the refinements in carbohydrate milling. These days, most snacks consist of sweet and sticky foods. Kids eat foods like cakes, muffins, and cookies very often, which is why dental caries' prevalence has increased.

Many studies show that sugars have a decay-promoting effect locally on the tooth surface. Starchy food, such as bread, is not as *cariogenic* as sugar. The amount of sugar ingested is not as important as the frequency with which someone snacks. Nowadays, it seems like everybody snacks more than they eat meals. If a snack is sweet and/ or sticky, and it stays on the tooth, then the bacteria in the mouth has more time to break the snack down into acid. The longer that acid is in contact with the tooth surface, the more damage it will do and the more cavities it will create. In contrast, if the food is easily washed down or rinsed away, less damage to the tooth surface and less cavity formation will follow.

NURSING BOTTLE CARIES

Sometimes a mother or caretaker will put a baby to sleep with a bottle in the infant's mouth. If the bottle is filled with milk, the sugars in that milk will break down into acid that will cause cavities. Anything that has got juice or honey and goes in the mouth (especially if it goes into the mouth during sleep, when the salivary glands are not as active) can cause tooth decay called *nursing bottle caries*. This caries is rampant, meaning it involves many teeth, and is quick in progression. It is important that parents and caretakers know they should give nothing but water to children at bedtime.

EFFECT OF DIET ON TOOTH DECAY

Some studies show that the kinds of diets people eat actually change the bacterial flora in their mouths, which can change the amount of cavities they get. A low-carbohydrate diet will reduce all the bacteria that cause cavities, and it will increase the protective bacteria. If a child eats a low-fat, high-carbohydrate diet during tooth development, then adding just a small amount of sugar can make that child's diet highly cariogenic (that is, causing caries). A high-fat, low-carbohydrate diet would require the addition of much more sugar to become cariogenic.

At our practice, when my colleagues and I meet a patient with rampant tooth decay, one thing we examine is that patient's food habits. Often, we suggest that the patient should keep a food diary for five days. During that time, he or she should write down exactly what he or she has eaten as specifically as possible; in other words, he or she should not just note generalities like "juice," but determine what kind of juice and how much juice. If he or she eats chicken, for example, he or she has to include how it was prepared and how much of it he or she ate. The patient gets the diary back to my colleagues or me when he or she comes back in for a follow-up appointment. My colleagues or I will go over the diary with the patient and make him or her notate all the food products containing sugar. This includes sugar added to a product and food that is naturally sweet, like fruit. Then, we ask the patient to try to cut down on these foods by slowly changing his or her diet.

People develop food habits very gradually from infancy through childhood, and these habits are not easy to change. Such change depends on what kind of food supply an individual had when he or she was growing up; his or her family's eating practices; and his or her social customs and educational influences. Many different things create people's food habits. Adult food habits are not easily altered because such habits are very deeply entrenched. An adult is adaptable only when he or she accepts that a change has to be made and that he or she will reap an advantage from making that change. Evolution, not revolution, is the guiding principle in modifying food habits. People cannot just say, "Let's take off the muffins and the cookies. We are going to go on a celery-and-carrot diet from now on." Such drastic change is not going to happen.

In treatment, we focus first on what is good in a patient's dietary habits, and then we encourage that patient to expand into eating other things that he or she can accept. We try to negate the cariogenic foods by increasing the good foods. We do not tell a patient, "Don't eat cookies"; instead, we tell him or her, "Eat so many portions of fruit." After that, we hope the patient will be so satisfied by the fruit that he or she will not want the cookies. Dietary change has to be conducted slowly. A saying by Mark Twain applies here: "Habit is habit and not to be flung out of the window by any man, but coaxed downstairs a step at a time."

What is Nutritional Deficiency?

Nutritional deficiencies are very complex. A single nutrient does not work by itself. It works with a combination of other nutrients. It carries out its function(s) along with adequate supplies of many other, related nutrients. Therefore, in many instances, when a person has a nutritional deficiency, he or she does not just have a single nutritional deficiency; he or she has more than one. Different nutrients interact and work together for optimal food metabolism and stability in the body; for instance, a vitamin B complex is required for the metabolism of carbohydrates, which ultimately provides organisms with energy. If a person eats more carbohydrates and has less of the vitamin B complex, this deficiency is going to show up as a carbohydrate deficiency in that person's body because the carbohydrates are not being metabolized. Proteins are metabolized with riboflavin, which also is part of the vitamin B complex; as a result, protein deficiency is matched by riboflavin deficiency. However, when a dentist looks in the mouth of a patient and sees different symptoms, it is not easy for him or her to pinpoint what nutritional deficiency is being presented by those symptoms. In such a case, the dentist will refer the patient to a physician for testing. Dentists can help patients figure out if the latter's symptoms are due to local irritant factors or, possibly, systemic nutritional deficiency.

Types of Nutritional Deficiency

There are two different kinds of nutritional deficiencies or nutritional inadequacies. The first type, malnutrition, is caused by faulty selection of food, and it is referred to as *primary nutritional deficiency*. This deficiency could be related to any of the following: lack of knowledge of what an adequate diet should be, due to different fad diets or just poor food habits; very finicky food likes and dislikes; unavailability of proper foods; or just inadequate funds to buy food.

The secondary type of nutritional deficiency is brought about when a body is not healthy enough to ingest, digest, metabolize, or utilize the nutrients in food. This is a systemic disorder in the body itself. Potential causes could be any of the following: infection, nausea, vomiting, different allergies to different things, neurologic disorders, poor dentition, colitis, diarrhea, celiac disease, liver or gallbladder disease, chemotherapy, diabetes, or alcoholism. The cause of this systemic disorder could also be something that interferes with the digestion of food, like a gastrectomy or stomach-stapling related to weight loss.

EFFECTS OF NUTRITIONAL DEFICIENCY IN THE MOUTH

A deficiency usually begins with a very gradual tissue depletion of a particular nutrient. There are different levels of deficiency. The deficiency starts off as biochemical, with just a drop in the actual level of nutrients. Then the deficiency becomes physiological; in this stage, the function of the tissue or organ is impaired, but at this point the deficiency is still reversible. Finally, prolonged deficiency causes anatomical changes, which means there is an actual change in the structure of the tissue. In many cases, such a change is irreversible.

At our office, when my colleagues and I see a person's nutritional status, the first thing we do is collect data from them. We note the patient's complaints and his or her medical and social history. We do a dietary history and evaluation, which consists of the food diary or the journal described earlier. We do a physical examination and note if the patient has signs of obesity, anorexia, and so forth. After that, a colleague or I will look into the patient's mouth to check for anatomical or physiological changes.

Common symptoms of nutritional deficiencies include the following: weakness and fatigue; loss of appetite; loss of weight; painful, bleeding gums; sore lips, tongue, or oral mucous membranes; diarrhea; chronic nervousness: irritability: loss of ability to concentrate; confusion; memory loss; dizziness; lethargy; loss of manual dexterity; pains in the legs; and skin problems. The most common symptom in the mouth is a burning sensation on the tongue or the roof of the mouth, and this particular symptom is caused by irritation of the nerves. The causes for these symptoms overall could be innumerable and range from iron deficiency, folic acid deficiency, and B12 deficiency to uncontrolled diabetes or some kind of allergy.

Some color changes are apparent more quickly in the mouth because the skin is opaque while the mucous membrane in the mouth is not. If there is any change in an individual's vascularity, it is easier to note it in the mouth, since paleness in the mouth is more easily visible than on the skin. If a person is pale in the mouth, his or her condition could be caused by anemia. *Cheilosis,* or *cheilitis,* also known as *angular stomatitis*, shows up as inflammation and infection in the corners of the mouth. The causes for this condition are many, but commonly include metabolic disturbances, like deficiencies in riboflavin, niacin, vitamin B12, protein, or iron. Fungal infections can cause similar kind of symptoms, too.

The tongue is very sensitive and swells when it is infected. Loss of taste or enlarged papillae on the tongue, a coating on the tongue, and serration along the lateral edge of the tongue are symptoms that relate to a number of different systemic health problems.

Dental plaque causes local irritation and gingivitis, but nutritional deficiencies can cause the gums to react more severely to dental plaque than normal.

Conditions including more of a breakdown of tooth structure or gum tissue in a patient, or more of a breakdown of the patient's vascularity (as shown by easily bleeding gums), could be caused by deficiency in vitamin C.

The last step through which we can confirm nutritional deficiency is via lab tests run by a physician. Depending on the findings, a dentist or physician will initiate vitamin therapy or diet counseling for the patient.

> Note that over-nourishment exists just as nutritional deficiency does, and both contribute to an unhealthy body. Just as there can be malnourishment issues caused by taking in fewer vitamins and fewer nutrients, an important cause of dental caries or obesity is the higher frequency of eating. Through overeating, people can get too-high doses of vitamins, too, which can cause toxicity.

NUTRITIONAL COUNSELING FOR THE DENTAL PATIENT

While nutritional counseling is not for every dental patient, undergoing such counseling is very beneficial for a patient who wants to be informed about why he or she is getting dental caries and how he or she can prevent recurrent tooth decay around old fillings or help make his or her restorations last longer. Other oral symptoms can point to a patient's current, undesirable food selections and eating habits; such a patient can be referred to a nutritionist in order to improve his or her diet. Nutritional counseling is for patients who believe, care about, and give a high priority to preventative dentistry, and for patients who are willing to make ongoing efforts in improving their dental and overall health.

Along with making healthy diet changes, such as lowering the intake of carbohydrates and sugars, dentists can fight the causative bacteria of dental caries in other ways. Dentists can use anti-bacterial rinses, anti-bacterial varnishes, and fluoride varnishes that lower bacterial count on our patients. These methods will help lower the breakdown of the food into acid.

People already know the link between oral and systemic health; in particular, there is a well-known link between inflammation, *oxidative stress*, and systemic disease. This is an important area of interest in medicine right now because oral infection and periodontal disease, both risk factors, are basically inflammatory in nature. They also cause oxidative stress.

What Is Oxidative Stress?

When there are too many free radicals or *oxidants* in the body, the imbalance is called oxidative stress. In the mouth, oxidative stress is associated with infection of the gums and other soft tissue. However, there are other elements that also cause oxidative stress in the mouth:

alcohol consumption; exposure to nicotine; and even dental procedures that use bleaching agents, dental cement, or fillings. Oxidative stress in the oral cavity can contribute to systemic oxidative stress, which leads to chronic diseases, like rheumatoid arthritis, or vascular diseases, like heart attacks or strokes.

ROLE OF ANTIOXIDANTS IN REDUCING OXIDATIVE STRESS

A *free radical* is an unstable molecule. It starts with an unpaired electron. In a process called *oxidation*, an unpaired electron steals the electron from another molecule and creates a new, unstable free radical. Free radicals are also called oxidants because they cause oxidation. They increase in number because they are unstable. They try to make themselves stable by grabbing electrons from other molecules and making them unstable in turn.

Some free radicals occur naturally in the body, but they increase because of a variety of reasons: environmental and lifestyle factors, like stress, pollutants, and poor diet; other substances, like nicotine, alcohol, and substances in the oral cavity; and other dental materials and procedures. *Antioxidants* are the molecules that counteract the process of oxidation. They bond with the unpaired electrons of free radicals and neutralize the oxidation process so there is no need for those free radicals to get paired up with electrons. Most of the time, antioxidants can be found in fruits and vegetables. The newest developments in antioxidant supplements are topical antioxidants. Researchers are using topical antioxidants in people's mouths to neutralize free radicals in oral tissue and counteract the effects of smoking and pollution.

When dentists do any kind of dental procedure, like extract a tooth or do a filling, and when there is bleeding and/or trauma to the tooth or the soft tissue, there has to be a period of healing. The presence of free radicals, oxidative stress, pollutants (like tobacco), and even stress impair that healing. When dentists use antioxidants in patients' mouth to counteract the effect of these oxidants, the dentists get rid of those free radicals, protect the oral tissues, and hasten the healing of wound.

Diet and health are clearly connected, and nowhere more so than in the mouth. In this area, a patient, not a dentist, is in the driver's seat. It is not enough to go blindly to the dentist every six months, get one or two fillings done, and think that is all you need to do to take care of your teeth. A healthy diet is going to affect more than just an individual's teeth; that diet is going to affect the person's overall health in the long term.

CHAPTER SIX

AESTHETICS AND DENTISTRY

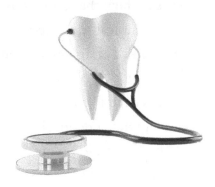

THE FIELD OF COSMETIC DENTISTRY, WHICH IS FOCUSED ON AESTHETICS, generally includes any dental work that improves the appearance, not necessarily the function, of a person's teeth, gums, and/or bite. Cosmetic dentistry is focused on creating beautiful smiles through addressing the color, form, and proportion of teeth.

The shape and length of the teeth are not one-size-fits-all. The shape of an individual's face and the squareness of his or her jaw make a big difference as to what shape and size of teeth fit into that face. The proportion of the teeth should suit a specific person, even his or her personality, not just the mouth.

Aesthetics is subjective because everybody has a different opinion about what looks good and what an attractive smile looks like. Each of us is influenced by touched-up photographs in magazines that show flawlessly white, straight teeth.

At one point in time, a patient could only guess what the outcome of a cosmetic procedure would look like. These days, dentists have technology available to show "before" and "after" pictures of a patient before doing anything to the teeth. Dentists can also make wax mock-ups of teeth models to show changes in teeth shape and size in all three dimensions. Having a realistic expectation of the cosmetic procedure greatly lessens the risk of disappointment for the patient.

There is not an established field of cosmetic or aesthetic specialization approved by the American Dental Association. For specialties like orthodontics or endodontics, a dentist has to go back to school and study that field specifically for a few more years. There is no such specialization required in order to practice cosmetic dentistry. There are many continuing education courses to which dentists can go in order to increase their knowledge, but attending is strictly elective. Any general dentist can say, "I'm a cosmetic dentist," and be able to do cosmetic dentistry. Therefore, it is up to the patient to ask for information and dig in to the level of education and experience of the selected dentist. Ask specific questions:

- What is your philosophy in cosmetic dentistry?
- How invasive or irreversible is this procedure?
- What are the risks involved?
- How am I going to know what I am going to get at the end of this procedure?
- Can you show me the "before and after" results?

Get more information before you jump right in and say to your dentist, "Give me that Hollywood smile."

Besides general dentistry, there are predominantly two dental specialties that deal with dental aesthetics: prosthodontics and ortho-dontics. A *prosthodontist* is the person who primarily does crowns and bridges. If a practitioner has to change the shape and size of a patient's teeth, not just the shade, then the practitioner has to add on to the teeth, either with bondings, crowns, or veneers. That, too, is part of the prosthodontic practice of dentistry. An *orthodontist*, or dentist who is trained in orthodontics, can straighten teeth. A big part of cosmetic dentistry deals with having straight, white teeth. A straight smile, one with no crowding or crookedness, comes from orthodontic treatment.

Cosmetic dentistry involving the addition of dental materials to either the teeth or gums bonding, adding porcelain veneers or laminates, performing crowns, and doing gum grafts are techniques involving addition to original teeth and gums.

VENEERS, CROWNS, AND BONDINGS

Simple bleaching cannot solve some teeth issues, such as the dimensions of the teeth, the shape or form of the teeth, or bleach-resistant stains. In those cases, dentists must use veneers, full-coverage crowns, or bondings to address any issues. Of the three possibilities, bondings are probably the least invasive because they use a composite filling. They also do not last very long. Bonding is not temporary, but it is not a permanent solution, either. A longer-term solution is the veneer, which will last almost as long as a crown. Early in their development, veneers were not as strong as they are now; they were basically just laminate material that dentists bonded onto the tops of teeth. Back then, veneers were made of composite material or porcelain gel.

These days, people use more porcelain to make veneers, as opposed to composite material, because the composite tends to get stained. Bondings will also stain because the matrix of the material is softer; it is not as resistant to stains. There are small micro-pores in the material that will absorb the stains, just like tooth structures. Porcelain does not pick up stains at all. It is very uncommon for porcelain to stain over a period of time, which is why porcelain veneers are longer-lasting. Crowns are done for cosmetic purposes only, such as when an individual really needs to change the major dimensions of the teeth. Dentists also advocate for crowns in cases when the teeth are already so worn down and cracked that an individual needs protection so that his or her teeth do not break; in such instances, crowns are used instead of veneers because veneers are not as protective a restoration as crowns are. A crown will cover the entire tooth structure. It will hold it all together; in contrast, the veneer only bonds to the facial aspect of the tooth in order to cover that tooth.

Bonding is a process in which an enamel-like dental composite material is used over the tooth surface, sculpted into shape, and then hardened and polished. The composite material used is somewhat porous, which can lead to eventual discoloration and staining. Although dentists now have some good materials to use that do not stain as much as other, older materials, these composite materials do not have the hardness of porcelain, so they can eventually crack.

IMPLANTS VERSUS FIXED BRIDGES

Let's talk about dental bridges or false teeth here because they too are part of cosmetics, especially in the front of the mouth. If a patient has a missing tooth in the front of the mouth, a dentist can do either implants or bridges. In bridges, the false teeth are called *pontics*. They are used to fill areas left by the missing teeth, and the two crowns that hold the bridge in place are attached to the adjacent sides of the false tooth. This is called a *fixed bridge*. This procedure is used to replace one or more missing teeth, and the resulting bridge cannot be taken out the way a partial denture can. In areas of the patient's mouth that are under less stress, like the area near a front tooth, a dentist might use a *cantilever bridge*, a bridge in which only one side of the tooth is crowned and the other side is the fake tooth. Instead of using two teeth, this process uses just the one tooth adjacent to the missing space. Dentists used the cantilever bridge procedure more commonly twenty years ago than today; now, dentists are more likely to replace a tooth either with a single crown and an implant or, sometimes, a regular bridge, depending on what is going on with the tooth next to the space.

Bridges can reduce the risk of gum disease and, sometimes, can help correct some bite issues. Having a bridge can even improve an individual's speech, since front teeth are very important for speech. If the front teeth are missing, a person will lisp. A bridge lasts a long time: five years, ten years, or even more. I have seen bridges last thirty years. The duration of the bridge depends on the patient, largely, and the environment of the mouth. A bridge does require commitment to serious oral hygiene, since one cannot floss a crown or bridge as easily as natural teeth; a bridge is a fused unit upon which the adjacent tooth and the fake tooth in the missing space are connected. One has to use floss threaders or different kinds of floss to go under the bridge and clean. If an individual does not do this, he or she can get gum issues, as well as tooth decay in the bridge area. In contrast, it is much easier to maintain an implant because the owner of the implant can still floss every individual tooth. An implant is not dependent on an adjacent tooth; in that way, it is less invasive. In addition, it is easier to clean around an implant. This is why dentists at my office recommend implants much more often for single tooth restorations, as opposed to bridges.

Let's go a little more in depth on the subject of veneers, which are ultrathin, custom-made, porcelain laminates. Bonded directly to the teeth, they can accomplish many different things. They can close gaps or disguise discolored teeth that do not respond well to whitening. Depending on the procedure and what kinds of changes an individual needs, a tooth reduction to accommodate the veneers may or may not be necessary. If an individual's teeth are already protruding, the dentist will have to reduce those teeth to accommodate additional material there. The decision depends on where the teeth are spatially in the mouth; however, these days, whenever possible, dentists are leaning toward prep-less veneers. These veneers require just two appointments; at the first one, the dentist takes an impression and sends it to the lab, where lab technicians make the veneers. The patient comes back a few weeks later, and then the dentist bonds those veneers onto the teeth. This is a fixed method; the veneers are bonded to the teeth and they do not come off. While the veneers can be removed, to do so the dentist has to remove both the bonding materials and the cement. This is not a simple procedure to reverse.

Snap-On Smile™

The Snap-On Smile™ is a patented, easy, and painless way to obtain a beautiful smile. A dentist who realized that not every person could afford to spend thousands of dollars to get the full Hollywood-smile makeover invented it. The Snap-On Smile™ is thin and strong, and it looks like a set of natural teeth. You can eat and drink with it on, and caring for it is easy. This method is completely reversible because the teeth are not altered at all. The Snap-On Smile™ is removable, not bonded onto the teeth. A Snap-On Smile™ can be a total solution, or it can be used temporarily to show a patient what his or her teeth will look like after a more permanent solution, like bonding. When delivering a Snap-On Smile™, the dentist takes an impression of the patient's mouth in an initial visit, and then he or she delivers the Snap-On Smile™ at the next patient visit. This method is completely functional, and the Snap-On Smile™ can be used in place of a partial denture in order to restore missing teeth. It is not as permanent as putting in veneers, but it is definitely more affordable. A whole Snap-On Smile™ will probably cost as much as just one or two veneers. It is not something that will last forever; a Snap-On Smile™ lasts for perhaps three to five years. The Snap-On Smile™ is not made of porcelain, but of dental resin. Still, the great appearance it can offer at an affordable price can give a person back confidence in his or her smile, which can be a life-changing experience. There is, of course, no drilling, no shots, and no change in tooth structure, which is always a good thing. The Snap-On Smile™ is an excellent choice for people who have gaps, crooked, stained, or missing teeth; for those who are not candidates for bridges or implants; or for anyone who would like to have a great smile without the expense or discomfort of invasive dental procedures.

The most basic advance in cosmetic dentistry has been the development of white fillings and bondings. These days, very few people get silver fillings. The materials that dentists use now are mostly all tooth-colored, even for back teeth.

GUM GRAFTS

Gingival recession (root exposure by loss of gums at the neck of the teeth) may be caused by exercising abnormal forces on teeth such as clenching or grinding, by practicing abnormal brushing techniques, or by experiencing gum disease. It is also a part of aging. The best way to cover the exposed roots is by using a gum graft. There are other ways of covering the exposure, for instance, bonding to the root surface, but that usually gives a more elongated appearance to the tooth, which is not very proportional to the mouth. Gum grafts are a big part of cosmetic dentistry. Generally, periodontists perform these, but some general dentists do grafts also.

TECHNIQUES INVOLVING REMOVAL OF TOOTH STRUCTURES AND GUMS

An example of the removal of tooth structure in cosmetic dentistry is when a dentist performs *enameloplasty* or *odontoplasty*, which is redefining or restructuring the teeth by removal. A *tooth reshaping*, which involves removing part of the enamel to improve the appearance of the tooth, can be done to correct a small chip or alter the length, shape, or position of the tooth. Tooth reshaping can be used to correct even crooked or excessively long teeth. This technique is called, variously, *enameloplasty, odontoplasty, contouring, recontouring, slenderizing, stripping,* or *sculpting.* This procedure offers a very fast result. It can even be substituted for braces in certain circumstances, such as when the teeth are just a little bit crooked, by reshaping the teeth and making them look straight.

Enameloplasty may sometimes expose dentin, which can cause sensitivity. That is why, the majority of the time that I do enameloplasties, I do not numb a patient because I am expecting him or her to tell me when to stop. If he or she feels any amount of sensitivity, I stop; the sensitivity indicates I am exposing too much dentin. At that point, I will put some kind of re-mineralizing material or desensitizer over the tooth, so the dentin is protected.

The removal of gum tissue is called a *gingivectomy.* This procedure works well when the teeth are too short and the smile is too "gummy"; that is, when the smile presents a great deal of gum exposure. In some cases, a dentist is able to take off some of the gum because the tooth has not erupted fully and there is still gum covering it. This procedure does not expose the roots; instead, it exposes more teeth, which makes the root-to-crown ratio better. A gingivectomy can be done either by surgery or by laser contouring of the gums.

STRAIGHTENING TEETH BY ORTHODONTICS

Straightening and aligning teeth may be accompanied by improvement in the appearance of the face, since changing the alignment and angulation of teeth can change the facial profile. Surgical correction is required if a person has a class III appearance (in which the chin is predominant compared to the upper jaw) or a class II discrepancy (in which the upper jaw is protrusive compared to the lower jaw), and the situation is a skeletal discrepancy, and not dental or teeth related.

Crooked teeth are a common problem, and everybody wants to straighten them if they can. There are many different ways of moving teeth or straightening teeth with today's new orthodontic technology. In order to find the right method of teeth straightening for every patient's specific circumstances, each patient needs to start with a consultation with the dentist. Nowadays, it is not just orthodontists who do braces; there are general dentists who do it, too. Getting braces is becoming more affordable and it is becoming faster. Patients are not necessarily stuck with old-style metal braces, either; instead, people can choose among clear braces, lingual braces, and porcelain braces. There are different kinds of clear alignment trays that are nearly invisible when worn. What each person needs depends on the kind of crowding in the mouth and the amount of tooth movement that is required. Alignment trays have improved so much that now these aligners can unravel any kind of tooth crowding.

Orthodontics is no longer, of course, just for a younger age group. I have treated people seventy years old and older who are straightening their teeth. People come to realize how crooked teeth can affect their bite, can affect their TMJ, and can affect their whole body. Straight teeth even help with nutrition because they enable more effective chewing and contribute to better oral hygiene. When an individual has crooked teeth and a protruded jaw, the tongue falls back, which can actually lead to sleep apnea. Expanding the jaw and getting more space for the tongue will help that individual to sleep better and can reduce the risk of sleep apnea.

The many different situations in which braces can be used lead to a plethora of different types of treatment. Dentists can change just the alignment of the front teeth, if that area is where the problem lies. Dentists can provide Six-Month Smiles™ and Fastbraces™. There are different ways of cosmetically aligning the teeth without changing an individual's bite.

On the other end of the spectrum, such as cases in which children have a skeletal discrepancy that will lead to excessive teeth crowding and other potential issues, dentists can intervene early and effectively with orthodontics. When a child grows up into adulthood, those issues are much harder to correct, whether skeletally or orthodontically. It is much easier to put in an expander for a few months, when a child is eight or nine, as opposed to doing years of orthodontics and skilled surgery on adults. Here are a few questions that a parent should always ask a dentist when taking a child in for an exam: how the child's teeth are doing in terms of spacing and alignment, if the child needs expanders, and if there are any signs that habits like sucking the thumb are having negative impact on the child's mouth.

CLEAR ALIGNERS VERSUS CONVENTIONAL BRACES

Let's go over the advantages and disadvantages of braces as opposed to clear plastic alignment trays. Dentists tend to give the alignment trays to adults or to teenagers over the age of fourteen. These trays are not for children; they are only for responsible adults and teenagers because using a tray requires a great deal of patient compliance. These alignment trays have to be changed every two weeks, and that change is the patient's responsibility. The patient has to be responsible for not losing the trays, too. The patient cannot eat or drink with the trays in, so a patient may take the trays out and then forget them somewhere. Consistency in wearing the trays is very important; they need to be worn almost 20 out of 24 hours in a day. People should only remove the trays in order to eat, drink, and change at the right time. If that protocol is not followed, then the teeth are not going to move.

Regarding braces with conventional brackets, whether those braces are clear, lingual, or metallic, they are fixed on the teeth. This means the patient does not have to be responsible in the same way.

Once the braces are put in, the patient will come in to the office every five to six weeks for a follow-up appointment; at that time, the dentist will change the wires or the elastics. With this system, the dentist is looking at the movement of the patient's teeth much more consistently than he or she would be doing with the aligners. Of course, the major advantage of aligners is that a patient can maintain really good oral hygiene while using them. The patient can take the trays out and floss, brush, and keep his or her teeth sparkling clean in between tray changes.

I have noticed that people who have aligners have better oral hygiene than they did when they were not wearing the aligners; this could be because people do not want to put the aligners on dirty teeth. Doing so does not feel good. Brackets, braces, and wires – all that stuff that braces put in the mouth – do not allow for good oral hygiene. Even the most fastidious patient will have some gingivitis and some plaque retention around the brackets, just because it is hard to clean or floss. That is the major disadvantage of braces.

Gums can be an issue in cosmetics, as previously mentioned. A gummy smile is not too attractive. It can be an issue that needs to be treated with laser recontouring, or it can cause a situation in which the lip is traveling up too high when an individual smiles. Some dentists will put Botox in the lip so the lip does not travel as high. I myself do not perform this; however, I have seen the results, and using Botox leads to a drastic change. The lip line suddenly becomes right over the teeth, so that now the individual has teeth in the smile instead of gums.

Another challenge in restoring an aging smile is restoring vertical dimension. With aging, when an individual loses the length of the teeth through attrition and wear, the vertical dimension of the face will also be reduced. The nose and chin will tend to meet, and that will cause deepening of the line around the angle of the lips. That gives an individual a markedly aged appearance, and this can even happen to a young person. If an individual has lost vertical dimension because of grinding, that person can look 50 when he or she is 35. Restoring this loss of dimension can change facial profile drastically and vastly improve appearance.

The easiest way to increase the vertical dimension in a smile is by adding structure to those lengths. Adding structure can be done with crowns, a bridge, or, if the person has no teeth, dentures. Some dentures are known as "facelift dentures" because they make their wearers look and feel like they got facelifts. With this lift, the vertical dimension is suddenly restored, and all those deep lines around the face, the lips, and the nose disappear. The patient regains the height of the lower third of the face, which gives back that youthful look.

TEETH WHITENING

The whitening or bleaching of teeth is one of the most common cosmetic dental procedures. There are many different whitening options available, and more appear in the market every day. These options range from a wide range of over-the-counter products to office-based, dentist-supervised treatments. Besides the shape and size of the teeth, color is the most important part of the cosmetic appearance of the tooth. Tooth whitening is one of the most popular forms of cosmetic dentistry. As well as being the least invasive and the most budget-friendly, it can produce an almost instantaneous result, depending on the option an individual chooses. White teeth make a person look younger. People can get in-office whitening in one hour or purchase an over-the-counter home kit that can be used over several days. Most people will see a moderate to substantial improvement in the brightness of their smile, but maintenance of that brightness will require touch-ups over time. Such methods do not offer a permanent solution.

BLEACHING VERSUS WHITENING

The FDA defines *bleaching* and *whitening* very differently, even though people use the terms interchangeably most of the time. *Bleaching* usually refers to whitening teeth beyond their natural color; it uses products that contain hydrogen peroxide or carbamide peroxide. *Whitening*, in contrast, is restoring a tooth's color by removing debris or extensive stains. Even toothpaste can be a whitener. Whitening or stain-removing toothpastes, which may be a little more abrasive, do not have bleaching materials in them. I am going to use the terms *whitening* and *bleaching* interchangeably in explaining how the process works.

WHY DO TEETH NEED BLEACHING OR WHITENING?

Enamel, the outer layer of the teeth, is a *hydroxyapatite crystal,* which is a protein matrix impregnated with crystals. Some soft tissue and some hard tissue make up enamel. Microscopically, enamel has little gaps or rods in its structure. With age, the enamel gets worn down. Inside the enamel is the dentin, or the inner layer of the tooth, which is much more yellow than the enamel. When the enamel gets worn down with age and becomes more transparent, it shows more dentin, which reveals more yellow. In addition, tiny micro-cracks naturally occur in the enamel. These micro-cracks retain stains from foods and drinks. This retention of stains also causes a tooth to change its shade and get darker over time. While teeth whitening removes those stains and that debris, the cracks eventually fill up again.

Two types of stains can occur on teeth: extrinsic and intrinsic. An extrinsic stain appears on the surface of the teeth because of an individual's diet, usually because of the following: exposure to dark-colored beverages, like tea, coffee, or red wine; exposure to dark-colored foods, like mustard, soy sauce, ketchup, and so forth; and exposure to tobacco or nicotine. Most superficial extrinsic stains are minor and can be removed with brushing or dental cleaning and polishing. Over time, they get more stubborn, so they need to be bleached or whitened with some kind of bleaching agent. These extrinsic stains can also be incorporated into the tooth's inner layer or dentin. Over a period of time, if an individual does not do regular maintenance and does not have good oral hygiene, those extrinsic stains become harder to bleach out.

Intrinsic stains are a bit different. They are not superficial; they are usually ingrained in the interior of the teeth during tooth development. This could occur by exposure to medication, like tetracycline, or excessive ingestion of natural fluoride in water, which causes fluorosis. Intrinsic staining can also be caused by trauma to the tooth in childhood or even adulthood. When a person receives trauma on a tooth, the trauma leads to internal bleeding of the tooth's pulp. That blood gets into the microscopic, tube-like structures of the dentin. The blood oxidizes there, which darkens the tooth color. At one time, people thought intrinsic stains could not be treated by bleaching at all and that the only options were veneers or bonding: that is, adding some kind of opaque layer over the tooth to cover the stain. However, these days, sometimes a long-term bleaching treatment can remove even the deepest-set intrinsic stains. Of course, a dentist must supervise this kind of bleaching.

The biggest cause of teeth staining is age. As the teeth get worn down, they get darker. Teenagers have teeth that can be bleached the most easily. When people reach their twenties, their teeth have gotten a little yellower, although they are still easy to bleach. By the time people hit their forties, their teeth have gotten browner, and have incorporated more stains, so they need more maintenance. After hitting the fifties, if an individual has never bleached, and he or she has extrinsic stains that are so deeply ingrained they are almost intrinsic, the stains become much more stubborn. It takes longer to bleach them and to maintain a lighter shade of teeth.

The starting color of the teeth, of course, is very important. If an individual has white teeth that have changed shade or gotten darker over a period of time because of extrinsic issues, then that is easier to deal with than an individual who began with a less-white shade of teeth. Dentists cannot fight genetic predisposition very effectively. In the latter case, the individual's teeth could be made whiter, but they would not become as white as those of a person who had extrinsic stains but began with very white teeth. Another issue is the transparency or thinness of the enamel, since during this process the dentist is bleaching out enamel, not really bleaching out the dentin. Genetically speaking, again, if a person has thick, opaque enamel, his or her teeth will appear lighter and be more responsive to bleaching. Thinner, more translucent enamel shows dentin more and it is harder to bleach.

Eating habits are very important when it comes to maintaining lighter shades of teeth whiteness. Consumption of red wine, tea, coffee, soda, carrots, oranges, soya, mustard, and ketchup – anything that is either a very dark or a very bright shade – will cause staining over a period of years. In addition, consumption of many acidic foods, like citrus or vinegar, will cause enamel erosion. The enamel will become more transparent, and the inner layer of dentin will show through.

Other things that affect teeth coloring include smoking, grinding, and trauma. Smoking leaves brownish deposits that are easily absorbed into the tooth structure and cause staining. Grinding and trauma cause additional micro-cracks and more worn-down enamel; that, in turn, usually causes darkness in teeth coloring and leaves stains more toward the ragged edges of the teeth, where the teeth are worn down. Persons who grind will have and keep more stains.

TYPES OF TEETH WHITENING

Of the three major options for teeth whitening, in-office whitening is probably the quickest. Benefits appear in a short period of time. In-office whitening involves the very careful use of a high-concentration peroxide gel, which the dentist applies to the patient's teeth after protecting the gums with a painted-on layer referred to as a *paint-on rubber dam*. The dentist has to protect the patient's gums completely in order to make sure that the high-concentration gel does not touch any soft tissue. Because of the strength of the gel, this practice has to be done in the office. The practice has to be supervised by a dentist or a hygienist; different states have different laws regarding who can apply it. The gel must be applied every 15 minutes, either with or without the use of laser or zoom light. The practice can be performed using different lights, although it is also possible to do the procedure without the light. The total time period is 45 minutes to an hour.

After that, the dentist or hygienist provides follow-up instructions and a bleaching kit for the patient to use at home, so that the patient can continue bleaching for the next seven days if he or she wishes, following the in-office bleaching. The effects of this bleaching are very rapid and dramatic; it is possible to change the shade of the teeth almost two to nine shades in the office, which is pretty drastic.

Patients who have sensitive teeth should have a desensitizing treatment before receiving a bleaching treatment in order to prevent discomfort afterwards. It is very common for a patient who comes in with worn-down or cracked teeth to have issues with hot and cold sensitivity, since he or she will likely have more exposed nerve endings in the dentin. In such cases, my colleagues or I would give the patient a desensitizing gel to use for ten days before bleaching, thereby offsetting that sensitivity both during and after the bleaching time. Increased sensitivity after bleaching is one of the most common complaints I hear from patients. While it is just temporary, it can still be pretty uncomfortable. A patient gets "zingers," which are like flashes of spontaneous hot, shooting pain on the teeth. Desensitizers go a long way to solving the problem, which is why, when a patient goes home after doing the in-office bleaching, my colleagues or I give him or her desensitizing paste to use. I also tell such patients to refrain from consuming certain kinds of food and drink because the bleaching has just opened up all the teeth's enamel rods, cleaned them up, and bleached them, so they are very easy to fill up again. The worst thing a person can do after bleaching his or her teeth is to drink a glass of red wine. An individual who has just bleached his or her teeth has to be very careful to stay away from anything food or drink that is colored for at least a couple of weeks, so that the enamel rods do not absorb that stain. Over a period of time, the individual's saliva and fluoride in the toothpaste he or she uses will remineralize the enamel and seal the teeth off so those rods are no longer open and ready to accept all stains that quickly. Ten to fourteen days after the bleaching, the individual can go back to eating normally – but he or she has to understand that diet was the root cause of the staining. Therefore, the more he or she continues to consume colored food and drinks, the quicker he or she will need maintenance and touchups.

The second way to bleach teeth is with a professionally dispensed take-home whitening kit. There are lots of different products, but effectively they are all the same. They either use carbamide peroxide or hydrogen peroxide to bleach the teeth. With carbamide peroxide, an individual can dispense a higher concentration over the teeth because when the compound breaks down, it ultimately becomes a lower concentration of hydrogen peroxide. This is just a safer method of dispensing peroxide. Hydrogen peroxide is the active bleaching material; the hydrogen peroxide breaks into oxygen, which is what finally breaks the stains. That is the way the bleaching occurs. Take-home bleaching kits have lower concentrations of peroxide gel compared to the in-office kits. An individual using a take-home kit puts gel on the teeth and leaves it there for 30 minutes to an hour, or even overnight. The dental team crafts custom-made bleaching trays from a mold of the patient's teeth. Those trays are used to carry the gel to the mouth and keep the gel in contact with the teeth. The trays are necessary to make sure that the gel stays on the teeth in a uniform layer and does not extrude over to the other soft tissues, where it can cause tissue damage or burns. That is why, at my office, we always recommend professional whitening kits with custom-made bleaching trays, not the over-the-counter kind. The thermoplastic materials used in the latter, which require the patient to heat the molds and then press them over their teeth to make them conform, just do not fit as well. If a patient does not know how much bleach to put in or is not able to get the tray on the right spot, he or she can actually do damage to soft tissue.

Over-the-counter teeth whitening kits that do not require the use of a tray are the least expensive and most convenient. Usually, these kits are what I would recommend to a teenager. These kits come in the form of strips or paint-on pens, and the bleaching substances are much less concentrated than those in professionally dispensed take-home whiteners. The strips may not whiten an individual's entire smile uniformly, because their components are small. They are folded over the teeth, and the area they cover depends on the size of the teeth. Sometimes, a user can just do a few front teeth. These kits can also leak into the mouth and taste bad, or can be ingested by accident. Again, the materials in these kits have a very low concentration of bleach; they are not as high in risk as the other kits, but they are also not as effective.

Teeth whitening is subjective, like any other cosmetic dentistry practice. An individual interested in the process has to get a realistic idea from the dentist of how white his or her teeth can get, how long it will take to make those teeth white, and how long they can stay white. In some cases, even the dentist is not able to answer all those questions; the answers can differ from patient to patient because of genetics, diet, and the amount of extrinsic and intrinsic stains already present in the mouth. Often, it is hard to predict how quickly and how much an individual's teeth can be bleached.

At our office, my colleagues and I use shade guides, hand-held guides that show different shades of teeth coloring. We will match the shade to a patient's teeth before and after the bleaching process to measure the progress. The bleaching kits permit a difference between two shades of up to nine shades, which is a very wide range. While the range of results is hard to predict, we can tell patients that yellower teeth usually bleach better than bluish gray teeth. Then, depending on how long the stains have stayed on the teeth, the bleaching process can take longer or there could be more follow-up appointments. All these things are important to discuss beforehand because both the dentist and the patient want to avoid disappointment; the patient needs to know how realistic his or her expectations are and what he or she can expect with the results.

Safety Issues with Teeth Whitening

Teeth whitening is safe, as long as the procedures are followed as directed. The most common side effect of teeth whitening is sensitivity to temperature or to pressure. A few people experience spontaneous sharp, shooting pains; dentists can usually control such problems with desensitizers, either before or after the bleaching is done. Patients who have gum recession, major cracks in their teeth, or having leaking fillings will be more likely to have sensitivity. Dentists have to make sure a patient's teeth and gums are healthy before beginning bleaching, since the bleaching agent should never go into an active carious lesion. The agent should not be in touch with gums that are puffy, red, and bleeding. While many marketing campaigns out there are selling people on the ease of teeth bleaching, patients cannot get their teeth bleached until their teeth and gums are healthy. If that is not the case, they will have to get other work done before they can get their bleaching.

Dentists prescribe sensitivity toothpaste that contains potassium nitrate for patients to desensitize their teeth before and after bleaching. If the teeth are already sensitive, the patient should use this toothpaste for ten to fourteen days before bleaching. Gum irritation can be a side effect of bleaching, when the dentist is not able to isolate the gums well while bleaching.

Another issue that comes up sometimes is what we call "Technicolor teeth," or different shades of teeth. A patient needs to know that materials in the mouth – anything that has a bonding, veneer, or crown, or any kind of composite white filling – will not respond to bleach; only the tooth structure can be bleached. If a patient has bindings, veneers, and crowns right next to the teeth that he or she wants to bleach, a shade difference will result. Clearly, people do not want different shades on the same tooth or different shades right next to each other in the mouth, even if those shades are on different teeth. Once an individual bleaches his or her teeth, those restorations might need to be changed to match the bleached teeth.

Newly bleached teeth do need maintenance. An individual with such teeth should avoid dark-colored foods and beverages; if that person wants to drink a dark-colored liquid, he or she should drink it with a straw. At my office, we recommend good oral hygiene: brush, floss, and rinse the mouth right after consuming dark-colored food or liquid in order to remove the potential staining source as soon as possible. One important thing to note is that there is a lag time of almost two weeks after bleaching in order to stabilize the shade. When an individual has an in-office bleaching, his or her teeth can continue bleaching for the next few days. The shade takes a little time to stabilize. Recessed gums where the roots are exposed cannot be bleached. They have to be grafted or be covered by a restorative material. Note, too, that pregnant and nursing women should avoid teeth whitening. While there are no long-term studies on the effects of the chemicals, there is no reason to take such a risk.

THE CONTROVERSY OF
SILVER FILLINGS

Medical scientists are constantly revising their opinions in terms of how to best treat various conditions, and dental conditions are certainly no exception. Along with change, invariably areas of controversy erupt; one of these areas is the topic of silver fillings versus composite fillings, which has garnered enough attention to be worth discussing here.

First of all, let's talk about the two materials. What we call *silver filling* composition is mainly an amalgam: an alloy of mercury with various metals, like silver, copper, and so on, included. Once it is mixed or titrated, the amalgam will set to form a hard, restorative material that has a fairly good amount of compressive strength and wear resistance. It has lasted for years in patients' mouths. Along with gold, it is one of the oldest restorative materials in dentistry.

Composite filling material is a little bit harder to explain. In definition, it is a high-molecular-rate monomer that, when cured, creates a rigid, cross-linked polymer. There are different ways to cure this material. It is initially soft and doughy in consistency; either it cures on its own, through the process of a chemical cure, or it can cure through light. Most composite materials used as fillings in dentistry are made of light-cure material. The dentist shines a blue light on it, and that is how the filling material becomes hard. Again, the composite has a good amount of strength and is resistant to wear. Some fillers are added to this composite to increase its strength, resistance to wear, and ease of handling, as well as its shade. The fillers can be quartz, zirconia, or glass silica along with barium, strontium, or other materials. The filler is what gives the composite material its high amount of strength. The amount of filler and the kind of filler that a dentist puts in the composite can be adjusted to make the material either better for the back teeth or better for the front teeth, depending on whether the dentist wants it to be highly polished and glossy or just wants to strengthen it. (People chew with the back teeth, so those should be stronger).

Mercury is a liquid metal also known as *quicksilver*. The heavy silvery element is the only metal that remains liquid at standard conditions of temperature and pressure. It is a unique metal in that sense, and that is why dentists can use it to amalgamate other solid metals. Then, when it becomes an alloy, it sets up a compound as something solid and strong. One of the major things you should know about silver fillings, aside from whether or not such a filling is safe in a patient's mouth, is that disposing of these alloys or amalgams makes for an environmental hazard. Most of the people who are anti-amalgam say that if you cannot throw something out in the garbage and it is not safe to put in the ground, then it probably is not safe in a person's body, either. Many anti-amalgam people and organizations consider silver fillings the cause of a whole host of medical problems: damage to children's brains, kidneys, and immune systems; neurological problems and gastrointestinal problems; sleep disturbances; concentration problems; memory disturbances; lack of initiative; restlessness; and even Alzheimer's disease.

Some studies show that people's mercury absorption from silver fillings is four times more than the absorption rate from fish consumption, which is the only other real substantial amount of mercury consumption that can happen in the human body. Absorption of mercury from fish consumption is why women are told to avoid eating fish during pregnancy. It stands to reason that if people are avoiding fish because of the mercury in it, they probably should not be getting silver fillings that will release four times the amount of mercury into their bodies, especially if there is an alternative available.

Canada will very likely ban silver fillings in the near future. Many countries in Europe have already done so. In Sweden, Norway, and Germany, for instance, dentists cannot use silver fillings that contain mercury at all. For some reason, the United States still has very strong lobbies supporting silver fillings.

Mercury builds up in the organs – especially in the brain, kidneys, and liver – and passes to infants through breast milk. It can also deposit itself in the pituitary glands and the adrenal glands. The thing about this particular metal is that it does not excrete out of the body as much as other substances; it deposits itself in the organs and it stays there. There is a cumulative effect as the mercury releases slowly, over years and years; as dentists add more and more silver fillings in a patient's mouth, the effect increases. Again, the decision about whether to use silver fillings is a matter of risk versus what one may have available as an alternative. If there is a safer alternative, common sense says that the safer alternative is what you should select. Formerly, gold was the only other alternative, but it was expensive and not static enough. Silver fillings were more available and cheaper. Today, because of the composite, which is the plastic matrix with the fillers, dentists can make a filling that is almost as strong as porcelain and that provides a natural appearance and better wear; plus, this material is obviously safer. Even apart from reducing the dangers of mercury exposure, selecting a composite filling is a better way to go for restoration in the cases of both children and adults.

Composite fillings have other advantages, too. For instance, composite fillings bond to teeth. They do not require the removal of tooth structure for mechanical retention, so they are less invasive and, of course, they are aesthetically far superior. Traditionally, silver fillings require a boxed preparation. The dentist makes undercuts in the tooth and then packs the silver filling in so that it locks into the tooth. This is a mechanical retention; those undercuts will lock the filling in, which is what makes the filling stay in the tooth. This process requires removing a great deal more of the tooth structure; in addition, the filling itself acts as a wedge in the tooth, since the tooth is more flexible than the silver filling material. Ultimately, this causes the tooth to fracture around the silver filling. When that happens, again, more tooth structure is lost. Sooner or later, the individual with the silver filling is likely to need to replace that tooth with a crown. In contrast to silver fillings, composite filling will bond to the tooth, requires much less removal of the tooth, and can stay forever without needing restoration. Even if the composite does break or crack, the dentist can simply take out the patient's composite filling and replace it with another filling; doing so does not crack the teeth. The composite material has actually been shown to increase the strength of even a cracked tooth because it bonds the tooth together instead of wedging it apart. There are no undercuts required, nor is there a big box required for use when putting in the composite filling.

Silver fillings do break down, and they do need to be replaced. Some holistic dentists will tell you that in the process of removing the silver filling, the mercury vaporizes and the patient can ingest or inhale the mercury. These dentists use suction instruments and masks when removing such fillings. Ordinary dentists simply drill out the silver filling and replace it. Of course, these dentists use suction instruments to make sure that the patients are not swallowing the fillings, but they do not use special techniques or equipment.

The scientific approach to silver fillings and their health effects is by no means settled. The American Dental Association does not believe that silver fillings cause any health issues. If a dentist removes a patient's silver filling because the filling is causing a health issue or because the filling is exposing the patient to mercury, the American Dental Association would consider such a removal ethical malpractice. Removal of silver fillings by a patient's request, because of aesthetics, because the filling is leaking, or because there is decay and the filling is breaking are all considered sound, acceptable reasons for replacement.

Significantly, the other big pro-amalgam organizations are insurance companies. Many of these companies will not cover composite fillings, although some of them do. They will cover silver fillings; so, basically, their policies encourage people to have silver fillings. If a person can get a silver filling for free, but must pay out of pocket for a composite filling, he or she will most likely want what is free. Personally, I do not think an insurance company should be the authority on what is best for a patient or dictate treatment options. A patient should think about his or her health, first and foremost, and then decide on what he or she wants.

WHY ARE COMPOSITE FILLINGS MORE EXPENSIVE THAN SILVER FILLINGS?

Composite fillings are more sensitive to the dentist's technique. The materials, by themselves, are more expensive. The steps in placing the materials in a tooth require more meticulous handling, and it takes longer to place them than it does to install silver amalgam fillings. Still, in my opinion, even if you take out the mercury factor, the benefits of using a composite filling far outweigh the cost; if you are anticipating that the silver fillings may need crowns later on, you are also anticipating paying five times the fillings' cost in the end, regardless. There are alternatives; many dentists today advertise themselves as "metal-free" practitioners. Be sure that you understand your dentist's philosophy before you go into treatment, and determine whether or not that philosophy agrees with yours.

CHAPTER SEVEN

ALTERNATIVE IDEAS TO DENTISTRY

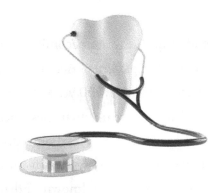

MANY DENTISTS ARE ADDING SOME FORM OF ALTERNATIVE DENTISTRY to the conventional, traditional dentistry that they studied in school. Nowadays, some schools are starting to add classes on topics in alternative dentistry as adjunct materials to conventional dentistry. Alternative therapies can be very helpful for some patients, especially patients with chronic head and neck pain, or those who have symptoms of TMJ disorder. Alternative dentistry is a good idea for areas in which conventional dentistry does not really offer a solution – for areas in which there is nothing medically that dentists can see or fix.

ACUPUNCTURE AND ACUPRESSURE

Acupuncture and acupressure are becoming increasingly popular as sources of pain relief for patients. Acupuncture is not new, of course; it has been used for some 3,000 years. It originated in China, where it has been used to treat many maladies, including infectious diseases, musculoskeletal diseases, metabolic diseases, hormonal imbalances, and mental and nervous system disorders. Over the last 50 years or so, it has become better known and more accepted in Western countries. There is a vast quantity of research documenting the idea that acupuncture is effective and safe. It is not voodoo. It has some scientific basis, even though it does come from traditional Chinese medicine. Often, when a patient has acute or chronic pain that is difficult to treat with conventional resources, acupuncture can be beneficial. Acupuncture has both an anti-inflammatory effect and an analgesic effect. It can help muscles relax. It has basal regulatory effects, which means that it can increase blood circulation in certain areas. It also has a sedative effect and an endocrinological effect. Acupuncture is done with fine needles placed in different *meridians*, or at different points on the skin that, according to Chinese medicine, increase energy flow, or *Chi*, in those areas. Chinese medicine practitioners believe that blockage in an individual's *Chi* can cause inflammation and pain, and that acupuncture can help create better energy flow. Applying controlled pressure to these points is called acupressure. In dentistry, acupressure can be used for pain management, reducing anxiety, increasing muscle relaxation, and providing anti-inflammatory effects.

The University of North Carolina School of Dentistry uses acupuncture for management of pain in orofacial pain clinics. Their representatives state that dental acupuncture can manage jaw pain or GMD, jaw ticking or locking, chronic muscle pain or spasms, tension headaches, migraines, nerve pain, neuralgia, neuropathic pain, nerve injuries, prominent gag reflex, dental anxiety, and xerostomia. Dentists can use acupressure points to increase salivation, which can reduce the amount of tooth decay in a patient's mouth. Sometimes, a patient can experience a burning sensation in the mouth or tongue, a sensation that can be eased with acupuncture. Another way to use those meridian points to treat pain is through the application of heat, or *moxibustion.*

Whether a dentist is using needles, heat, or pressure, he or she is stimulating the nervous system. It changes the way we process pain signals and releases natural painkillers, such as endorphins and serotonin, in the nervous system; that is the Western way of explaining *Chi.* The response to treatment varies from immediate improvement to requiring several treatments to get the full benefit to not benefiting or responding at all. According to the Traditional Acupuncture Association, 70 percent of the patients who receive treatment have some benefit. Providing relief to about 70 percent of patients who are in pain, who have no other relief, and have tried everything else, is a huge accomplishment.

Pain in muscles is usually characterized by local *ischemia* (decreased blood supply in that area), inflammation, and accumulation of toxins. Increasing blood supply helps to flush away toxins faster. This lowers inflammation and hastens healing.

Acupressure or acupuncture helps people in two different ways. One is in the local area that has caused the pain. Another is in distant areas, called *projection zones*, which are further away from the origin of the pain. The Chinese call these zones meridians. When a practitioner applies pressure on an acupressure point, he or she can restore the local and projected symptom areas at the same time.

Practitioners apply acupressure or acupuncture to specific points for pain relief or for symptom relief, either around the area(s) of pain itself or through a corresponding meridian. For example, the pressure point located in the web of the hand, between the thumb and forefinger, is frequently used to help reduce pain or dental anxiety.

THE MODIFIED TENS UNIT

In our office, we use microcurrent therapy on acupuncture points. The therapy machine is classified as a modified TENS (transcutaneous electrical nerve stimulation) unit, and it works by sending tiny electrical impulses first to locate and then to stimulate both the patient's nerve and acupuncture point. When properly stimulated, the muscles affected by the trigger point relax. Muscle relaxation improves blood circulation and triggers the release of endorphins, which are natural painkillers produced by the body. The body's natural healing response is stimulated, and pain can be reduced in a safe, non-pharmacological manner.

Nerve points or trigger motor points are tiny, tight bundles of nerve endings that are located throughout the muscles. They become tender when related muscles get injured. These points on the skin display lower electrical resistance than the surrounding tissue. At our office, we use this shift in resistance to figure out where to direct the TENS unit, since the handheld device we use has a display light that switches off when it hits the right spot. It is very hard to take the TENS unit to the wrong spot on a patient because of the fact that the electrical resistance is different on that particular nerve ending. It is very precisely identified and stimulated, and the electrical impulse cause the physiological results of traditional acupuncture and trigger point needling, without the actual risks associated with using needles. This device should not be used on pregnant women, patients who have cancer, epileptics, or patients who have cardiac pacemakers.

The efficacy of the treatment is amazing. We saw 50 percent to 75 percent relief among our patients within the first four treatments. The TENS unit is tremendously helpful to individuals who have jaw pain. It can be used in other areas, too, including treatment of gag reflex and xerostomia.

HOMEOPATHY IN DENTISTRY

The next area of alternative dentistry I want to talk about is *homeopathy*, which is a system of healing that seeks to cure illness in accordance with certain principles of healing. Homeopathy utilizes remedies made from plants, minerals, and animal products. The practitioners prepare remedies according to a process of repeated dilution and shaking. The practitioners then direct treatment toward strengthening a person so that his or her own healing capacity can take care of his or her problem.

At our office, the way we treat a patient by using homeopathy is very different than the approach offered in traditional Western medicine. We find out the actual constitution of the patient; when he or she has pain in a certain area, what other sensations or symptoms accompany that pain? Does it make him or her feel cold and clammy? Does it give him or her hot flashes? Does it happen in the daytime or does it happen in the nighttime? Does it make him or her feel thirsty, or does it make him or her not want to drink water? There are many different symptoms that go along with that one primary symptom, and discovering them is what constitutional homeopathy is about. While we are treating dental disorders, by figuring out what the different systems associated with patients' primary symptoms are, we can use homeopathy to discover the main cause(s) of the disease through all the mental, emotional, and physical symptoms specified by the patient. By seeing the entire symptom, a practitioner can then treat the patient as a whole, rather than treating the disease as it presents itself locally. That is the basis of homeopathy.

Many people do not believe in homeopathy. They believe that it is total quackery. I was raised in a house where all our family's colds, coughs, fevers, and other ailments were treated homeopathically. Homeopathy is far more common in Eastern medicine than it is in Western medicine. As far as I know, there is no specific regulatory board that covers the practice of homeopathy in Texas, where my office is located. Homeopathy can be used for mild trauma, which patients experience on their gums and cheeks, or for abscess ulcers.

It can be used for anxiety. If our patients are open to it, we usually recommend it for discomfort after extractions, for discomfort after a deep cleaning, or for minor areas of trauma or abrasion. These patients are already more in tune with wanting to use something herbal or homeopathic, instead of using something more traditional. They would rather use a particular tincture to treat an area of abrasion than take an over-the-counter pain medication that could cause gastric upsets or drowsiness.

Homeopathic treatment can also provide relief for bruxism (teeth grinding), which is a very difficult problem to treat, particularly in children. Homeopathic treatment is also useful for xerostomia (dry mouth) and hyper-salivation. Some patients just have a great deal of saliva, which makes it hard to do dental work on them. In such cases, a homeopathic remedy given thirty minutes before an appointment can be beneficial for both the patient and the dentist. Conditions like these, along with others that we do not have great solutions for in conventional dentistry, like sore jaws after extensive dental work or dry sockets, can be treated by homeopathy

NOTE: Homeopathic medicine is not a substitute for antibiotics or other medications prescribed by a physician or dentist. It is useful as an adjunct to conventional medicine or in conditions when conventional medicine has failed.

HERBAL REMEDIES IN DENTISTRY

An *herb*, botanically speaking, is any plant that lacks the woody tissue characteristic of a shrub or a tree. More specifically, herbs are plants that are used medicinally, or for their flavors or scents. Herbs with medicinal properties are useful and effective sources of treatment of varied different diseases, and many drugs used these days in Western medical science have their origins in medicinal plants. Many people believe that herbal medicine or herbal supplements are much safer than allopathic, or Western medicine; however, it is important to know that herbal medicines have strong pharmacological effects and are not necessarily safer than other medications. People must be very careful in taking them. Herbal supplements like St. John's Wort, for example, or other over-the-counter medications sold in nutrition and vitamin stores can adversely affect a patient who is already on medication and create potentially dangerous drug interactions. That is why it is very important that a patient tells his or her dentist or physician what he or she is taking in supplements.

There are many herbal remedies related to dentistry. People often use calendula and echinacea to soothe gums and to reduce inflammation. These herbs are also effective in preventing *candidiasis* and other opportunistic yeast diseases in the mouth. Taking a calendula tincture diluted with equal amounts of water and swishing it in the mouth for several minutes is helpful for patients with periodontal disease. Lavender oil may be used to clear up many kinds of fungal infections or for reducing inflammation and healing sores. Goldenseal, oregano, and grapeseed are used in dentistry for their antimicrobial effects. Rosemary, which is used for gum sores, also has antiseptic properties. Parsley is a natural breath freshener, as is licorice. Aniseed is commonly used to freshen the breath after eating Indian food. Oil of cloves is a common remedy for toothache or for soothing the sore gums of a teething baby.

> **NOTE:** These remedies maybe used at home, but they still need to be discussed with a dentist first.

I do want to share a simple mouthwash recipe here: Take a teaspoon of rosemary (dried), a teaspoon of mint (dried), and a teaspoon of fennel seed. Boil two and a half cups of water, and pour the liquid over the herbs. Let the mixture steep for to 20 minutes. Strain and cool; then, it is ready to use.

Complementary and alternative medicine (CAM) represents a group of diverse medical and healthcare systems, practices, and products that are not considered part of conventional medicine. Biofeedback, acupuncture, herbal medication, massage, bioelectromagnetic therapy, meditation, and music therapy are all examples of CAM treatments. Some dentists in the United States have started to use some of these treatments and products in their practices. Complementary medicines include herbal remedies, homeopathic medicines, and essential oils. Over the last 15 to 20 years, there has been an increase in the use of herbal medicines in the U.S. There is a public belief that these medicines are safe because they are made from natural sources. However, some of these products have associated adverse effects including toxicity and drug interactions. The patient's health history taken by the dentist should include questions regarding the taking of herbal and over-the-counter medications.

A dentist needs to be informed regarding the herbal and over-the-counter products that may impact the delivery of safe and effective dental treatment.

CHAPTER EIGHT

THE TRUE MEANING OF HOLISTIC DENTISTRY

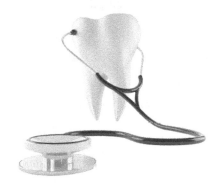

TO ME, HOLISTIC DENTISTRY IS REALLY ABOUT BEING W-H-O-L-I-S-T-I-C, since a dentist needs to do an evaluation of the whole body of the patient, not just his or her mouth. Dentistry requires an understanding of the connections between the mouth, the teeth, the gums, the oral cavity, and the rest of the body. I hope that in reading this book, the connections between the head and neck, and between the mouth and the body, have been made clear to you.

The primary rule for all healthcare providers is, first, to do no harm. It is important for both the patient and the dentist to understand that regardless of the influence of society or organizations, insurance companies, and so forth, a dentist has to be conscientious about what is being put in the patient's mouth. First and foremost, it should not be hazardous to the patient's health in any way. The next step is to benefit the patient in every way possible. Knowing the connections between the oral cavity, TMJ, the jaw relation, and the bite on body posture, the spine, the back, and even serious conditions like sleep apnea, it is the dentist's job, as a physician of the mouth, to screen patients for medical conditions and to refer them to the right medical professionals for early intervention and treatment.

Your mindset as a patient, when you go to the dentist and ask for your six-month checkup and cleaning, needs to change as you realize the importance of these screenings. The same thing goes for your meetings with a physician or specialists in the dental field. These professionals need to understand the dental and medical connection is very strong and requires better cross-referrals for better overall care of the patient. There are too many overmedicated patients, including children. Why does a physician give migraine medication or neuralgia medication, which has significant side effects, to a patient for 20-plus years without considering that this problem might have a dental perspective and might be a bite issue? Medical practitioners in all fields need to open their minds to issues beyond their immediate scope of practice. For instance, remember that there is a 70 percent overlap between grinding and sleep apnea. The doctor who is treating the sleep apnea, as well as the dentist who is treating the grinding, need to come together on that issue to help the patient. There has to be a point at which the dentist and the physician realize that the jaw, the mouth, and the whole of the body are all connected and part of the whole; what goes in the mouth can affect the body and vice versa.

A patient should be open to questions by the dentist regarding sleep habits, medication, anxiety, chronic pains, and the existence of other medical conditions. Much of the time, the patient just brushes over those questions, saying, "That's not important for you to know. You are just fixing my teeth." The patient should know that the focus of dentistry has shifted not just to treating the tooth, but also to treating the body via the teeth.

Indeed, dentistry has shifted to a less invasive, more diagnostic and preventive kind of dentistry. It is not about just fillings. It is about what causes that cavity. There is more risk assessment and more nutritional counseling. Dentists today use more preventative measures to prevent gum disease, screen for bacteria, and treat specific diseases with a specific treatment program. With better technology, knowledge, and materials, we are able to do more. These advances also make dentistry more comfortable and painless because early diagnosis and intervention means doing the least invasive dental procedures.

It is important for parents to know that the symptoms associated with ADD are also present in children who have sleep apnea. An expander is a type of treatment that can substitute for a lifetime of medication.

Regarding the latest trends in cosmetics, a patient should realize that there are many different, less invasive, and more natural-looking treatments available now. There are strong, all-porcelain crowns, as well as aesthetic materials for fillings to choose from, so that dentists can practice metal-free dentistry easily. It is not only more attractive but also more practical to do that; it lasts longer, and there are more predictable results. Many treatment options, from veneers to Snap-On Smiles™, allow a patient to restore or gain the confidence only a beautiful smile can bring. There is no reason to deny yourself that gift.

As an informed consumer, the patient needs to ask the dentist what his or her diagnostic skills are and what diagnostic technology is available in the office. The range is broad and extends from dentists who use no digital radiography to dentists who will do a saliva te before they try to treat gum disease because they want to know which specific bacteria is causing the problem. A whole array of different standards of dentistry is available, and the patient needs to know what is out there before making the choice of practitioner.

Today, the practice of dentistry is much more rewarding and exciting for both the practitioner and the patient; it is also much more comfortable. Dental phobia should really be a thing of the past. There are many new, different methods of relaxation, including non-pharmacological techniques for decreasing dental anxiety. As a result, any patient who has been avoiding the dentist for years because his or her memories of the last visit still results in nightmares, need fear no longer.

By ignoring dental treatment, you are not just ignoring your teeth; you are ignoring your body. You are putting yourself at risk for creating more dangerous health conditions that extend far beyond just having no teeth in your mouth.

As Dale Carnegie once said, "Keep your mind open to change all the time; welcome it, court it. It is only by examining and re-examining your opinions and ideas that you can process them."